Parasites, Pussycats and Psychosis

E. Fuller Torrey

Parasites, Pussycats and Psychosis

The Unknown Dangers of Human Toxoplasmosis

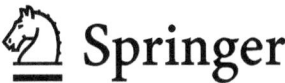 Springer

E. Fuller Torrey
Stanley Medical Research Institute
Bethesda, MD, USA

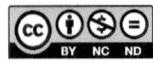

This book is an open access publication.
ISBN 978-3-030-86810-9   ISBN 978-3-030-86811-6   (eBook)
https://doi.org/10.1007/978-3-030-86811-6

This Springer imprint is published by the registered company Springer Nature Switzerland AG
The registered company address is: Gewerbestrasse 11, 6330 Cham, Switzerland

"In that direction," the Cat said, waving its right paw around, "lives a Hatter: and in that direction," waving the other paw, "lives a March Hare. Visit either you like: they're both mad."

"But I don't want to go among mad people," Alice remarked.

"Oh, you can't help that," said the Cat: "we're all mad here."

Lewis Carroll, Alice's Adventures in Wonderland

For Barbara, to whom I am indebted for 54 great years.

Preface

I like cats. They make nice companions, especially for people living alone. I won't say I like them better than dogs because that would seem disrespectful to the cocker spaniel of my childhood, very loving though not very bright. I became especially fond of Meowser, onomatopoeically named by the woman who lived next door who, when she went to work in the morning, let the cat outside. During the winter months Meowser learned that by climbing up on the porch furniture adjacent to my ground-floor study and looking at me sadly I would let her in for the day. She usually slept on the rug next to my chair, the heater under my desk being a major attraction, but on some days she would wander upstairs and stretch out on her favorite chair. I understand why writers such as Mark Twain, Ernest Hemingway, and Henry James have praised cats, the latter even claiming to have written with his cat lying on his shoulder. Being particularly well fed, it was clear that neither Meowser nor my shoulder were up for such a task.

Coincidentally, at the time Meowser was visiting I was writing a book, *Beasts of the Earth*, about how infectious agents spread from animals to humans and cause many human diseases. This book is about one such disease, toxoplasmosis, caused by a protozoa carried by cats. To be sure Meowser and her ancestors bear no responsibility for this. The protozoa probably infected feline ancestors several million years ago and simply found cat intestines to be the ideal place to complete its life cycle. In the course of evolving, the protozoa learned how to reprogram infected rat brains to increase the chances of the rat being eaten by a cat, thereby making it possible for the protozoa to return to a cat's intestine. As discussed in Chap. 2, the protozoa also learned how to reprogram the brains of red foxes, hyena cubs, chimpanzees, and who knows how many other animals. Since I am one of the 40 million Americans who is infected with the toxoplasma protozoa, perhaps it also learned how to reprogram my brain. Perhaps that is why I am writing this book.

Regarding the terminology used in this book, I use the terms madness, insanity, and psychosis interchangeably. Each has been popular at different times in history, but all imply a loss of contact with reality, marked by symptoms such as delusions and hallucinations. In contemporary clinical terminology these terms include all individuals with schizophrenia and schizoaffective disorder, a significant subset of those with bipolar disorder, and a smaller subset of those with major depressive disorder. Insofar as some cases of psychosis are caused by toxoplasmosis, it would open up vast new possibilities for treatment as well as prevention.

Bethesda, MD, USA   E. Fuller Torrey

Acknowledgments

I wish to thank Springer Nature for encouraging the publication of books such as this by open access. Medical research data should be available to researchers and clinicians worldwide. Richard Lansing, Cecily Berberat, and Anila Vijayan at Springer efficiently facilitated the publication of this book.

I am indebted to Robert Yolken, my friend and research collaborator for four decades. His research staff at the Stanley Laboratory for Developmental Neurovirology, Johns Hopkins University, has carried out much important research on *Toxoplasma gondii* and other infectious agents in relationship to serious mental illnesses.

Many thanks also go to Elisabeth Maselli and the Rutgers University Press and to Judy Miller, my co-author of *The Invisible Plague*, for permission to reuse some material from that book on the rise of psychosis in England.

Marie McIntyre at the University of Liverpool kindly shared with me the useful Enhanced Infectious Diseases Database (EID-2) created by her and her colleagues. I am also indebted to Jaroslav Flegr and to Joanne Webster for their important pioneering research on toxoplasmosis that has helped direct attention to human aspects of this disease. Vernon Carruthers, Robert Taylor, and Maree Webster provided very useful comments on portions of the manuscript. Shen Zhong kindly kept my computer and dictating system functioning well. And many thanks are owed to my research assistant, Wendy Simmons, who cheerfully and carefully carried out the myriad tasks associated with putting a book like this together.

Finally, I must thank the following for permission to use images of paintings in their collections to illustrate the changing social status of cats.

- The Recanti Musei, Recanti, Italy for Lorenzo Lotto's "The Annunciation"
- Angelo Tartufuri, Director of Museo San Marco, Florence, Italy for Domenico Ghirlandiao's "The Last Supper"
- The West Suffolk Heritage Service for Mary Beale's "Portrait of a Girl with a Cat"
- Victoria Art Gallery, Bath for Johann Zoffany's "Portrait of Sophie Dumergue"
- Leeds Museums and Galleries (Leeds Art Gallery) UK, copyright: Leeds Museums and Galleries/Bridgeman Images for Walter Crane's "At Home: A Portrait"
- The Clark Art Institute, Williamstown, MA, for Pierre Auguste Renoir's "Sleeping Girl"

Contents

About the Author

Dr. E. Fuller Torrey is a research psychiatrist specializing in schizophrenia and bipolar disorder and infectious agents as possible causes of these diseases. He holds degrees from Princeton (AB), McGill (MD), and Stanford (MA in anthropology) universities and trained in psychiatry at the latter. He is currently the Associate Director for Research at the Stanley Medical Research Institute and Professor of Psychiatry at the Uniformed Services University of the Health Sciences. He has authored or co-authored 20 books including *Beasts of the Earth: Animals, Humans and Disease* and *Surviving Schizophrenia*, now in its seventh edition. *The Roots of Treason*, his biography of Ezra Pound, was nominated as one of the five best biographies of 1983 by the National Book Critics Circle.

Other Books by the Author

- *Ethical Issues in Medicine: The Role of the Physician in Today's Society* (Boston: Little, Brown and Co., 1968). Edited and wrote two chapters.
- *The Mind Game: Witchdoctors and Psychiatrists* (New York: Emerson Hall, 1972)
- *The Death of Psychiatry* (Philadelphia: Chilton, 1974)
- *Why Did You Do That? Rainy Day Games for a Postindustrial Society* (Philadelphia: Chilton, 1975)
- *Schizophrenia and Civilization* (New York: Jason Aronson Inc., 1980)
- *Surviving Schizophrenia: A Family Manual* (New York, Harper and Row, 1983)
- *The Roots of Treason: Ezra Pound and the Secret of St. Elizabeths* (New York: McGraw-Hill, 1983)
- *Nowhere To Go: The Tragic Odyssey of the Homeless Mentally Ill* (New York: Harper and Row, 1988)
- *Frontier Justice: The Rise and Fall of the Loomis Gang* (Utica: North Country Books, 1992)
- *Freudian Fraud: The Malignant Effect of Freud's Theory on American Thought and Culture* (New York: HarperCollins, 1992)
- *Criminalizing the Seriously Mentally Ill: The Abuse of Jails as Mental Hospitals.* Senior author. (Washington DC: Health Research Group and National Alliance for the Mentally Ill, 1992)

- *Schizophrenia and Manic-Depressive Disorder: The Biological Roots of Mental Illness as Revealed by a Landmark Study of Identical Twins.* Senior author. (New York: Basic Books, 1994)
- *Out of the Shadows: Confronting America's Mental Illness Crisis* (New York: John Wiley and Sons, 1997)
- *The Invisible Plague: The Rise of Mental Illness from 1750 to the Present.* Senior author. (New Brunswick, N.J.: Rutgers University Press, 2001)
- *Surviving Manic Depression: A Manual on Bipolar Disorder for Patients, Families and Providers.* Senior author. (New York: Basic Books, 2002)
- *Beasts of the Earth: Animals, Humans, and Disease.* Senior author (New Brunswick, N.J.: Rutgers University Press, 2005)
- *Surviving Prostate Cancer: What You Need to Know to Make Informed Decisions* (New Haven: Yale University Press, 2006)
- *The Insanity Offense: How America's Failure to Treat the Seriously Mentally Ill Endangers Its Citizens* (New York: W.W. Norton, 2008)
- *The Martyrdom of Abolitionist Charles Torrey* (Baton Rouge: Louisiana State University Press, 2013)
- *American Psychosis: How the Federal Government Destroyed the Mental Illness Treatment System* (New York: Oxford University Press, 2014)
- *Evolving Brains, Emerging Gods: Early Humans and the Origins of Religion* (New York: Columbia University Press, 2017).

Psychosis as a Zoonosis: Clues from Covid

1

1.1 Diseases from Animals

This book proposes that an infectious agent may be transmitted from animals, specifically cats, to humans and then cause some cases of psychosis. As such, the thesis includes two major problems. First, most people do not think of infectious agents as being transmitted from animals to humans. Second, most people do not think of human psychosis, including diseases such as schizophrenia and bipolar disorder, as being caused by infectious agents. Thus we must first resolve these two issues before we can expect to make any headway on the overriding thesis.

Except for a few diseases such as rabies, we do not generally think of human diseases as being transmitted to us from animals. The Covid pandemic of 2020–2021 reminded us forcefully that such transmission can indeed take place with devastating consequences. The coronavirus which causes covid most likely originated in bats although it may have passed through other animals before reaching us.

In fact, it has been clearly established that the majority of human diseases are caused by infectious agents which have been transmitted to us from animals. Some of them were transmitted in the distant past, such as the hepatitis virus that we acquired from our primate forefathers in the process of evolution. Other infectious agents, such as the bacteria that cause anthrax and brucellosis, were transmitted to humans during our millions of years of hunting and butchering animals. During the agricultural revolution approximately 10,000 years ago, we domesticated a variety of animals and, in the process, acquired a variety of diseases. For example, it is suspected that we acquired the microbe that causes stomach ulcers from sheep, tuberculosis from goats, whooping cough from pigs, measles from cattle, glanders from horses, smallpox from water buffalo, typhoid fever from chickens, and influenza from ducks. We sometimes romanticize the past as having been more free of diseases than the present, but in reality the opposite was true. In the Garden of Eden, Adam may have had herpes virus cold sores, Eve may have had hepatitis, and the snake was almost certainly carrying salmonella bacteria [1].

© E. Fuller Torrey 2022
E. F. Torrey, *Parasites, Pussycats and Psychosis*,
https://doi.org/10.1007/978-3-030-86811-6_1

It is not only that human diseases were acquired from animals in the past; Covid has confirmed that the process is ongoing. In 2001 Scottish researchers listed 175 infectious agents known to cause diseases in humans. Of these, 132, or 75%, are known to be transmitted from animals. In 2004 the director of the Centers for Disease Control and Prevention (CDC) noted that "11 of the last 12 emerging infectious disease that we're aware of in the world, that have human health consequences, have probably arisen from animal sources." In summary, it seems very plausible that any disease affecting humans could have been transmitted from animals [2, 3].

1.2   Bats and Rats, but Please, Not Cats

The idea that bats or rats can cause human disease because of the infectious agents that they carry is one thing, but the idea that cats can be similarly responsible is quite another. In the United States, according to the 2010 census, 32% of house-holds owned at least one cat. The total number of owned cats in the United States is thought to total approximately 90 million. In addition, there are estimated to be anywhere from 30 to 80 million feral cats, with the Humane Society suggesting a median estimate of 50 million. That would put the total number of cats in the United States at 140 million; since there are estimated to be a total of approximately 600 million cats in the world, the United States would have almost one quarter of them.

Cats are not like bats or rats or other animals. In recent years their status has changed from being merely animals to becoming human companions. For example, in Colorado, legislation was introduced to change their legal status from "property" to "companion." In Mississippi a man petitioned the Department of Agriculture to allow him to use his food stamps to buy food for his pets. In Minnesota a company allows employees to take a week of "paw-ternity" leave and work at home when they acquire a new cat or dog. More than 30 states now require emergency officials to have plans for pet evacuations in disasters. Expenditures by American families on their pets in 2016 surpassed $60 billion, approximately the same as the gross national product of Afghanistan, Bolivia, Nepal, or Uganda [4–8].

One consequence of viewing cats as human companions rather than as animals is the intimacy it implies. Thus it has been reported that 75% of pet cats in the United States are allowed to sleep on the beds of their owners—62% on the beds of adults and 13% on the beds of children. In both England and France, 45% of cats sleep on their owners' beds, and in the Netherlands, the figure is 62%. Such intimacy makes it more likely that any infectious agent being carried by the cat will be transmitted to the cat's owner, and in fact studies have identified cases of bubonic plague, cat scratch disease, and other diseases that have been transmitted to humans by cats which slept with them [9].

As cats transitioned from being merely animals to becoming human companions in the latter half of the twentieth century and early years of the twenty-first century, cats experienced a profound increase in popularity. A harbinger of this change was Catwoman, who first appeared in the Batman comics in 1940. Initially, Catwoman was a villain, but by the 1970s, she had taken on a more nuanced role, occasionally acting as Batman's helper and even as his love interest. Catwoman drove a cat-illac and used a bullwhip as her weapon of choice. In the Batman movies of 1966, 1992, 2004, and 2012, Catwoman was played by Eartha Kitt, Michelle Pfeiffer, Halle Berry, and Ann Hathaway.

Another comic strip character that has popularized cats is Garfield, an orange, fuzzy tabby cat who debuted in 1978. Garfield is owned by Jon Arbuckle who also has a beagle named Odie, and it is with Jon and Odie that Garfield mostly interacts. Garfield represents human weaknesses insofar as he is overweight, eats too much (he is especially fond of lasagna), disdains any exercise or work, hates Mondays, and is self-centered. By 2002, Garfield had become the most widely syndicated comic strip in the world. This popularity was developed into multiple movies and television primetime specials, at least four of which won Emmy awards, as well as into a Saturday morning cartoon series. It has also spawned a variety of Garfield-associated merchandise, including clothing, toys, videogames, books, dolls, and credit cards. Other movies that helped to popularize cats include "That Darn Cat" (1965) and "Aristocats" (1978), which was the last film approved by Walt Disney prior to his death [10, 11].

A major advance in the promotion of cats was the musical by that name. Written by Andrew Lloyd Webber, it was based on T.S. Eliot's *Old Possum's Book of Practical Cats*. It opened in London in 1981 and ran continuously for 21 years, setting a record for being the longest running musical until it was surpassed by "Les Misérables." "Cats" opened in New York in 1982 and ran continuously for 18 years, also setting a record until surpassed by "The Phantom of the Opera." "Cats" has been translated into more than 20 languages and produced in 34 countries in addition to the United States. Rum Tum Tugger, Old Deuteronomy, and the other cats are now known worldwide, many having their own entry on Wikipedia.

Despite the popularity of cats achieved by comics, movies, and a musical, nothing has promoted the image of cats as much as the Internet. According to Wikipedia, as of 2015, there were over two million cat videos on YouTube and as many as 6.5 billion total cat pictures on the Internet. Indeed, cats have been said to be the "unofficial mascot of the Internet." An Internet celebrity such as "Grumpy Cat" had more than 20 million views of its original YouTube video and 4 million followers on Instagram and had its own agent who signed advertising deals. It was featured on the front page of the *Wall Street Journal* and, when it died in 2019, was given an obituary with picture in *The New York Times* [12–14].

Given this status, it is difficult to think of cats in the same category as bats and rats as carriers of infectious agents that cause human disease. But that is indeed the case. The most extensive work on this question has been carried out by Dr. Marie McIntyre and her colleagues at the University of Liverpool. They created a public database, the Enhanced Infectious Diseases Database (EID-2), that includes 273 infectious agents that have been identified in cats, of which 151 are known to be shared with humans. These include infectious agents causing diseases such as the following:

- *Viral*: cowpox, rabies
- *Bacterial:* anthrax, campylobacter enteritis, cat scratch disease, diphtheria, liste-riosis, Lyme disease, plague, salmonellosis, shigellosis, streptococcal infection, tularemia, yersiniosis
- *Rickettsial:* Q fever
- *Spirochetal:* leptospirosis
- *Fungal:* ringworm, blastomycosis, sporotrichosis
- *Protozoal:* amebic dysentery, giardiasis, toxoplasmosis
- *Worms:* hydatid disease, cutaneous larva migrans, visceral larva migrans
- *Arachnids:* scabies

Several of these diseases are serious and not uncommon; for example, 60 cases of cat scratch disease were diagnosed in the state of Connecticut in a 13-month period [15–17].

The fact that cats can become infected with the coronavirus that causes Covid disease is simply one more example of an infectious agent that can be carried by cats. And it was not surprising, given the fact that cats are known to be infected with a related feline coronavirus. During the initial Covid outbreak in New York City, it quickly became apparent that the cat family was susceptible to the disease when three lions in the Bronx Zoo were diagnosed with Covid, apparently having become infected by the zookeepers. Later it was shown that a tiger and a snow leopard were also infected. Since that time it has been shown that both cats and dogs can become infected, although both show only mild symptoms. In one study it was reported that in households in which a person was infected with Covid, 24% of the household cats and 15% of the dogs were also infected. It has also been shown that infected cats can pass the Covid virus to other cats. To date, however, there is no evidence that cats transmit the virus back to uninfected humans. This stands in contrast to the situation on mink farms where mink are raised commercially for their pelts; not only do mink become severely infected and even die from Covid, but they also have been proven to spread the virus back to humans. Because the virus was also mutating in the mink, causing concern that it might become resistant to the vaccines, the government of Denmark abolished all mink farming in that country [18–20].

1.3   The Origin of Cats

Cats in one form or another have been around for 25 million years. Thus they have had plenty of time to acquire infectious agents, some of which took up permanent residence. One such infectious agent is *Toxoplasma gondii* which will be discussed in the following chapter. Among the most successful early members of the cat family were saber tooth cats, one of which is incorrectly referred to as a saber tooth tiger. Modern tigers, along with leopards, jaguars, and lions, all evolved within the past 2 million years. Wildcats (*Felis silvestris*) also separated from the other felids about 2 million years ago. The European wildcat (*Felis silvestris silvestris*) spread widely across Europe, including the British Isles at the time when it was still connected to Europe by a land bridge. The European wildcat is now found only in sparsely inhabited regions of Europe, including Northern Scotland. The African wildcat (*Felis silvestris lybica*) was widespread in Northern Africa and Southwest Asia and is the only wildcat that has ever been domesticated. It can and does interbreed with European wildcats. Three other species of wildcats are found in Southern Africa and Asia.

Following the agricultural revolution approximately 10,000 years ago, the first farmers in Southwest Asia began storing grain which attracted rodents. The African wildcat was plentiful in that region and, attracted by the rodents, began hanging around the grain storage areas. The farmers, in turn, tolerated the wildcats since they were providing some protection for their grain. We speak of the wildcats as having become domesticated, but even today some people would argue that the term "domesticated cats" is a contradiction in terms. The important point is that the earliest relationship between cats and humans was a distant one with little direct contact. The relationship was probably similar to how we think of feral cats today.

After farming had become established in Southwest Asia, it slowly spread. Farmers reached Southeast Europe by 8000 years ago, Central Europe by 7000 years ago, and Great Britain by 6000 years ago. As they moved westward, the farmers encountered the original settlers, modern *Homo sapiens* who had migrated out of Africa about 60,000 years ago and reached Europe by 45,000 years ago, and the two groups intermixed. The African wildcats followed the migratory farmers to Europe and apparently became increasingly domesticated over time. This explains why the remains of what appear to have been domesticated cats have been found in Europe, including in South West England dated to 250 BCE, prior to the arrival of Roman soldiers and traders [21].

In addition to spreading westward from Southwest Asia, farming also spread south into Egypt, beginning about 6500 years ago. Since African wildcats were indigenous to Egypt, they also killed the rodents there, thus protecting the grain. Egyptians deified many animals, including the bull, ibis, and crocodile, so it is not surprising that they also deified cats. Egyptians also tamed many animals and kept them as pets, including monkeys and hyenas, so it is also not surprising that they tamed cats. Originally, the Egyptian sacred cats were associated with a minor local deity, Bastet, who was the goddess of fertility in Bubastis, a city in Lower Egypt. However, 2950 years ago, in the 22nd Dynasty, Bubastis was made the capital of Egypt, and Bastet, as a cat-headed goddess, became much more widely worshipped. Later, Bastet became associated with Isis who was one of the principal Egyptian deities. It was this association that ultimately led to a widespread belief that cats were evil and agents of Satan, as will be discussed in Chap. 3.

It should be noted that cats were not associated with evil in ancient Egypt. On the contrary, they were depicted in temple drawings as being part of the household, often sitting under a chair or being fed from the dinner table. Herodotus, who toured

Egypt 2500 years ago, "reported that Bastet's temple in Bubastis was the most attractive in the whole country and her annual festival the most joyous and popular." He also noted that "when a house was on fire the Egyptians were more anxious to save their cats than their property" [22, 23].

The importance of cats in Egypt was apparently unique in the ancient world. There is no mention of them in the Old or New Testament, and they played a minor role in ancient Greece and Rome. Cats appear occasionally on Greek vases and Roman mosaics, including a mosaic from Pompeii, now in the Naples Museum, depicting a cat hunting birds in the marshes. But for rodent control, the Romans preferred ferrets, and as pets they strongly preferred dogs. In his book *Classical Cats*, Donald Engels noted: "Many tombstones were erected by bereaved Romans to their pet dogs, but none are known for cats" [24].

1.4   Infectious Agents and Psychosis

The second major problem associated with the thesis of this book is that most people are unaware that psychosis can be caused by infectious agents. This is especially true for viruses. Herpes simplex virus, for example, usually causes cold sores around the mouth but occasionally gets in the brain and causes psychosis that may look identical to schizophrenia or bipolar disorder. Other herpes viruses, such as the cytomegalovirus and the Epstein-Barr virus, may also occasionally cause psychosis. One of the best-known causes of infectious psychosis is the influenza virus. During the pandemic of what was called Russian influenza in 1889–1892 and again during the pandemic of 1918–1919, cases of psychosis following infection were widely described in individuals who had no previous psychiatric history. Although viruses are the most common cause of psychosis among infectious agents, others can do so also. The spirochete that causes syphilis, for example, was said to be responsible for up to 10% of the psychosis cases in some psychiatric hospitals prior to the introduction of penicillin. The parasite *Toxoplasma gondii* can also cause psychosis, as will be described in the next chapter [25].

The Covid pandemic of 2020–2021, caused by a coronavirus, provided a dramatic reminder that infectious agents can cause psychosis as well as a variety of other psychiatric and neurological symptoms. Previous studies had shown that other coronaviruses could cause psychosis, so this development was not a total surprise. A report summarizing the first 42 cases of Covid-related psychosis concluded that "already it is clear that infected patients can exhibit a range of neuropsychiatric symptoms." There appeared to be no relationship between the severity of the Covid symptoms and whether or not the patient developed psychosis. A preliminary study from England reported that there had been a 10% increase in cases of new onset psychosis in 2020 compared to 2019. More definitive studies will be forthcoming and will clarify the true incidence of psychosis associated with Covid disease [26, 27].

Additional evidence suggesting that infectious agents cause some cases of psychosis comes from national case registers in the Scandinavian countries. One study found an almost fivefold increase in adult schizophrenia in individuals who had had a viral infection of their central nervous system as children. A second study reported a 60% increase in the risk of schizophrenia for individuals who had been hospitalized for any infection. Consistent with such findings are multiple studies that report evidence of inflammation in individuals with schizophrenia. Such evidence includes pro-inflammatory markers such as cytokines and c-reactive protein as well as evidence of microglial activation, all consistent with an infectious process [28–31].

Yet another suggestion that psychosis is associated with infectious agents comes from genetic studies. Among all the reported findings from studies of the genetics of schizophrenia, one finding stands out as the strongest. An area on chromosome 6 is known as the major histocompatibility complex (MHC) and encodes more than 400 genes. A major function of these genes is to regulate the body's immune response, including its response to infectious agents. In genome-wide association studies of individuals with schizophrenia, the activation of the MHC complex has been the single most prominent and replicated finding. This is the part of the genome that would be expected to be activated by an infectious agent. In summary, based on multiple existing studies, it seems plausible that an infectious agent can cause a brain disease such as schizophrenia [32].

Although infectious agents were probably the most common cause of cases of psychosis in history, they were not the only cause. Another cause was brain trauma. Hominins have been beating each other over the head with clubs for as long as hominins have existed, and studies have shown that one of the consequences of head injuries is psychotic symptoms. For example, a follow-up of men who sustained severe head injuries in the Russo-Finnish war, at the onset of World War II, reported that psychotic symptoms occurred in 5% of cases. Epilepsy, which can also be caused by head trauma, is another ancient medical condition that may exhibit psychotic symptoms, especially if the temporal lobe of the brain is involved [33–35].

As long as hominins have existed, there have also been periods of severe food shortages and consequent starvation. One syndrome associated with food shortage, specifically an insufficient intake of niacin, is pellagra which may include symptoms of mania, hallucinations, and catatonia. Another ancient food-related cause of psychosis is ergot poisoning caused by a fungus that may infect food supplies, especially grains. Its symptoms may include mania and psychosis; outbreaks often occur in epidemics as groups of people are exposed to a common infected food supply. In the Middle Ages, ergotism was well known and referred to as Saint Anthony's fire.

Infections of the brain, head trauma, epilepsy, pellagra, and ergotism were probably the most common but not the only causes of madness in history. Others include genetic diseases such as Huntington's disease and porphyria, primary or metastatic cancer of the brain, and endocrine disorders such as severe hypothyroidism, the symptoms of which are often referred to as "myxedema madness." In more recent centuries, additional medical causes of madness include infections such as advanced syphilis and exposure to toxins such as mercury used by hat makers, memorialized by Lewis Carroll's "Mad Hatter."

Is there any estimate of the number of cases of madness, based on these known causes, which one would expect in a given population? This number would of course vary depending on the social circumstances, being higher, for example, after wars and famines. But one estimate of the prevalence of madness in history concluded that there was approximately one mad person for every 2000 people at any given time, or 0.5 cases per 1000 population point prevalence [36].

Given this background, what do we find when we look for cases of madness in history? We find occasional cases scattered throughout ancient texts, beginning with Mesopotamian clay tablets 5000 years old describing a man beset by "mischief makers" and "other evil machinations" suggesting paranoid delusions. The Old Testament also mentions madness several times. Deuteronomy 28 warns that "the Lord will smite you with madness and blindness and confusion of mind" if you break the commandments. In Daniel 4 Nebuchadnezzar is described as having a period of madness, then recovering. And Ezekiel was said to have experienced both auditory and visual hallucinations [37].

Occasional cases of madness were also described in ancient Greece and Rome. The cause of madness was usually attributed to disturbances of the humors, as described by Galen, although it was acknowledged that the gods could also cause madness. Herodotus, a Greek historian, described King Cleomenes of Sparta who exhibited bizarre behavior and committed suicide. Plutarch, a Greek biographer, recounted the bizarre behavior of a man who pretended to be Alexander the Great and attributed it to madness. Horace, a Roman poet, described a man who spent much time sitting in an empty theater applauding actors on an empty stage. Celsus, a Greek philosopher, described three different kinds of madness. Madness was also used by Greek writers and playwrights. Homer had Ajax become mad and Odysseus feign madness. Euripides had Orestes, who was being pursued by the Furies, briefly experience delusions and hallucinations [37, 38].

In reviewing these descriptions of madness in ancient literature, two aspects stand out. First, most cases are relatively brief, accompanied by fever or other medical symptoms, and followed by recovery. The symptoms of the madness described are consistent with infections of the brain and other medical causes of psychosis as described above. Second, the total number of cases of madness described in ancient texts is relatively few. This was emphasized by Katie Evans and her Australian colleagues who conducted an exhaustive search of Greek and Roman literature from the fifth century BCE to the middle of the second century CE. The search resulted in what they called "a handful of descriptions of psychotic symptoms" [38].

Now that we have established that infectious agents can be transmitted from animals to humans and have also established that infectious agents can cause psychosis, we can proceed to examine *Toxoplasma gondii.*

References

1. Torrey EF, Yolken RH. Beasts of the earth: animals, humans and disease. New Brunswick: Rutgers University Press; 2005.
2. Taylor LH, et al. Risk factors for human disease emergence. Philos Trans R Soc Lond Ser B. 2001;356:983–9.
3. ProMED-mail. Avian influenza, human, East Asia. January 29, 2004.
4. Sink M. Colorado: pets as companions. New York Times, February 11, 2003.
5. Dewey C. Advocates petition USDA to extend food stamps to pets. Washington Post, January 24, 2018.
6. Brulliard K. How the chaos of hurricane Katrina helped save pets from the Texas floods. Washington Post, September 1, 2017.
7. Haag M. Company's new pet owners get 'fur-ternity leave. Washington Post, August 21, 2018.
8. Spending on pets surpasses $60 Billion. JAVMA News. https://www.avma.org/News/JAVMANews/Pages/160515g.aspx.
9. Chomel BB, Sun B. Zoonoses in the bedroom. Emerg Infect Dis. 2011;17:167–72.
10. Wikipedia, entry for Garfield. https://en.wikipedia.org/wiki/Garfield.
11. Vocelle LA. Revered and reviled: a complete history of the domestic cat. Great Cat Publications; 2016. p. 329.
12. Wikipedia, entry for Cats and the Internet. https://en.wikipedia.org/wiki/Cats_and_the_Internet.
13. Lopez C. Why is the Internet obsessed with cats? https://petlifetoday.com/why-is-the-internet-obsessed-with-cats/.
14. Victor D. Grumpy cat, online symbol of surly living, is dead at 7. New York Times, May 18, 2019.
15. Thanks to Dr. Marie McIntyre for providing an analysis of data from the Enhanced Infectious Diseases (EID2) database. The EID2 is an open-access resource developed by a group including M. Baylis (P.I), K.M. McIntyre and M. Wardeh at the University of Liverpool; for more information see https://eid2.liverpool.ac.uk.
16. Lappin MR. Feline zoonotic diseases. Vet Clin N Am Small Anim Pract. 1993;23:57–78.
17. Zangwell KM, et al. Cat scratch disease in Connecticut. N Engl J Med. 1993;329:8–12.
18. Halfmann PJ, et al. Transmission of SARS-CoV-2 in domestic cats. N Engl J Med. 2020;383:592–4. https://doi.org/10.1056/NEJMc2013400.
19. Bosco-Lauth AM, et al. Experimental infection of domestic dogs and cats with SARS-CoV-2: pathogenesis, transmission, and response to reexposure in cats. Proc Natl Acad Sci. 2020;117(42):26382–8. https://doi.org/10.1073/pnas.2013102117.
20. Fritz M, et al. High prevalence of SARS-CoV-2 antibodies in pets from COVID-19+ households. One Health (Amsterdam, Netherlands). 2021;11:100192. https://doi.org/10.1016/j.onehlt.2020.100192.
21. Driscoll CA, et al. The Near Eastern origin of cat domestication. Science. 2007;317:519–23. https://doi.org/10.1126/science.1139518.
22. Rogers KM. *Cat*. London: Reaktion Books; 2006. p. 11–2.
23. Zeuner FE. A history of domesticated animals. London: Hutchinson; 1963. p. 391.
24. Engels D. Classical cats: the rise and fall of the sacred cat. New York: Rutledge; 1999. p. 93.
25. Torrey EF. Functional psychoses and viral encephalitis. Integr Psychiatry. 1986;3:224–36.
26. Severance EG, et al. Coronavirus immunoreactivity in individuals with a recent onset of psychotic symptoms. Schizophr Bull. 2011;37:101–7. https://doi.org/10.1093/schbul/sbp052.
27. Watson CJ, et al. COVID-19 and psychosis risk: real or delusional concern? Neurosci Lett. 2021;741:135491. https://doi.org/10.1016/j.neulet.2020.135491.
28. Miller BJ, Goldsmith DR. Evaluating the hypothesis that schizophrenia is an inflammatory disorder. Focus (American Psychiatric Publishing). 2020;18(4):391–401. https://doi.org/10.1176/appi.focus.20200015.

29. Rantakallio P, et al. Association between central nervous system infections during childhood and adult onset schizophrenia and other psychoses: a 28-year follow-up. Int J Epidemiol. 1997;26:837–43.
30. Benros ME, et al. Autoimmune diseases and severe infections as risk factors for schizophrenia: a 30-year population-based register. Am J Psychiatry. 2011;168:1303–10.
31. Muller N. Inflammation in schizophrenia: pathogenetic aspects and therapeutic considerations. Schizophr Bull. 2018;44:973–82.
32. Corvin A, Morris DW. Genome-wide association studies: findings at the major histocompatibility complex locus in psychosis. Biol Psychiatry. 2014;75:276–83.
33. Davison K, Bagley CR. Schizophrenia-like psychoses associated with organic disorders of the central nervous system: a review of the literature. In: Herrington RN, editor. Current problems in neuropsychiatry. Ashford, Kent: Hedley; 1969. p. 113–84.
34. Shukla GD, et al. Psychiatric manifestations in temporal lobe epilepsy: a controlled study. Br J Psychiatry. 1979;135:411–7.
35. Achte KA, Hillborn E, Aalbreg V. Psychoses following war brain injuries. Acta Psychiatr Scand. 1969;45:1–18.
36. Torrey EF, Miller J. The invisible plague: the rise and fall of mental illness from 1750 to the present. New Brunswick: Rutgers University Press; 2002. p. 343.
37. Jeste DV, et al. Did schizophrenia exist before the eighteenth century? Compr Psychiatry. 1985;26:493–503.
38. Evans K, et al. Searching for schizophrenia in ancient Greek and Roman literature: a systematic review. Acta Psychiatr Scand. 2003;107:323–30.

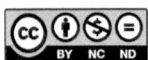

The Case for *Toxoplasma gondii* in Psychosis and Other Human Diseases

2

2.1 Modes of Transmission

This chapter introduces *Toxoplasma gondii*, the cause of toxoplasmosis. It discusses the many ways it can be transmitted and what is known about human infections, especially those affecting the brain, the pregnant uterus, and the eyes. It details the evidence linking this parasite to psychosis and estimates the percentage of psychosis cases that may be caused by it. It also briefly discusses the evidence linking toxoplasmosis to other conditions: epilepsy, brain cancer, rheumatoid arthritis, and motor vehicle accidents.

It has been called "one of the most successful parasites on Earth" and yet is one of medicine's best kept secrets. It is "remarkable in its ability to infect nearly any nucleated cell in any warm-blooded animal" and infects most species of mammals and birds. An estimated one third of the world's humans are infected although this varies widely by country, depending on dietary habits and exposure to cats. A 2014 survey in the United States reported that 11% of the population, or approximately 40 million Americans, have antibodies to this parasite indicating past infection [1–4].

For almost a century after its discovery, it remained largely unknown. It was given a tongue-twisting name, *Toxoplasma gondii*, which was in fact inadvertently misspelled—the North African rodent in which it was discovered in 1908 was a gundi, not a gondi. It is a protozoan parasite, not bacteria or viruses which were the infectious agents of greatest interest in the twentieth century. The most noteworthy protozoan is the malaria parasite; *T. gondii*, as it is commonly abbreviated, is a second cousin to the malaria parasite, but, like famous humans, second cousins don't get much press. It was not until 1938 that *T. gondii* was known to be transmitted from a pregnant woman to her fetus and to cause severe problems with brain development. And it was not until the late 1960s that cats were identified as the specific host for this parasite. *T. gondii* has to be eaten by a cat to complete its life cycle in the cat's intestine.

It begins its life cycle when a cat, usually as a kitten, becomes infected. Although the cat usually has no symptoms, it excretes in its feces up to 50 million infective

© E. Fuller Torrey 2022
E. F. Torrey, *Parasites, Pussycats and Psychosis*,
https://doi.org/10.1007/978-3-030-86811-6_2

T. gondii oocysts per day for an average of 8 days. At any given time approximately 1% of cats are infective and excreting oocysts. The oocysts are remarkably hearty and can survive for long periods in soil or water, as will be described in Chap. 7. Wherever the cat defecates may become contaminated with infectious oocysts. Since cats prefer loose soil for defecation, this often includes gardens, children's sandboxes, and animal feed piles in barns. After 24 hours the oocysts dry out and are thought by some researchers to become aerosolized, thus floating in the air and capable of being inhaled. Water becomes contaminated when cat feces deposited on the ground is carried into streams by rainwater or when cat litter is flushed down the toilet.

The variety of ways in which humans can become infected with *T. gondii* is impressive and not widely appreciated. Best known is the fact that pregnant women who become infected can pass the parasite on to their developing fetus, thus being an example of congenital transmission. For many years it was believed that a woman could only congenitally transmit *T. gondii* on one occasion. It is now known that at least occasionally she can become reinfected with a different strain of the parasite or become chronically infected. Similarly well known is the risk of becoming infected from contact with cat litter. However, it is usually not physical contact with cat litter that is the risk but rather breathing in the aerosolized *T. gondii* oocysts that may float in the air once the infected cat feces dry out. Therefore it is recommended that pregnant women not change cat litter. Recent studies have even identified *T. gondii* oocysts in the air near outside locations where cats frequently defecate. An outbreak of toxoplasmosis among 37 patrons of a cat-infested riding stable in Georgia was thought to have been caused by people inhaling the oocysts. Many people are also aware that one can become infected with toxoplasmosis by gardening or children playing in loose soil or sand in which infected cats have defecated. In one such outbreak, seven preschool-age children from an extended family in Alabama became infected after playing in sand piles which had been contaminated by infected cats. In another outbreak, four children from one family became infected with toxoplasmosis, presumably from exposure to infected family cats [5–9].

It is also reasonably well known that one can acquire toxoplasmosis by eating undercooked or raw meat. Many such outbreaks have been documented, such as five students in New York who all ate undercooked hamburger on the same night. Cows, sheep, pigs, and other animals become infected, for example, by eating animal feed in which an infected cat has defecated. *T. gondii* then develops cysts in the animal's muscle tissue that can infect humans if the meat is undercooked. Raw fruits and vegetables that have not been properly washed are additional sources of infection. In recent years, it has become clear that infected drinking water is also a major source of toxoplasmosis infection. Over 200 waterborne outbreaks have been documented, including 1 in Victoria, British Columbia, in which 100 people became clinically infected with toxoplasmosis [10–14].

Other possible modes of transmission of the *T. gondii* parasite to humans are still being explored. In a few cases, it has been passed on as part of an organ transplantation from an infected person. A recent study reported *T. gondii* infection in 2% of fleas from dogs and cats, raising the possibility that humans could become infected by petting them. A study of infectious agents left on the keypads of automated teller machines (ATMs) in New York City identified *T. gondii* on 1 of the 66 ATMs studied, perhaps left by someone who had been gardening prior to using the ATM. The possible sexual transmission of *T. gondii* is also under investigation; it has been shown to occur in dogs and sheep, and, since *T. gondii* oocysts have occasionally been found in the seminal fluid of men, it seems likely that sexual transmission also occurs in humans [15–19].

2.2   What Is Known Regarding Human Infections?

Given the fact that 11% of the American population is infected with *Toxoplasma gondii*, what symptoms do they have when they are infected? Fortunately in the vast majority of cases, they have very minor symptoms or no symptoms at all. For those who have symptoms, they are usually flulike, with fever, malaise, and often with enlarged lymph nodes. Such symptoms can be effectively treated with standard antiparasitic drugs. Thus most people who are infected with *T. gondii* are unaware that they are infected because doctors do not routinely test for it.

There are three major exceptions to this otherwise benign clinical picture. The first is cerebral toxoplasmosis. When *T. gondii* gets into the brain, it often causes major problems because we have no effective medications for toxoplasmosis that cross the blood-brain barrier and, thus, no effective treatments. Cerebral toxoplasmosis may affect individuals who are immunosuppressed, either because of having a disease such as HIV-AIDS or because of treatment for cancer or an organ transplant. For such individuals an initial infection with *T. gondii* or reactivation of the latent infection can result in severe toxoplasmosis, especially of the brain. Prior to the availability of effective treatments for AIDS, cerebral toxoplasmosis accounted for many deaths of these patients. Studies estimate a total of 1400 hospital visits and 71 deaths per year attributable to toxoplasmosis in the United States, two thirds of which are for cerebral toxoplasmosis [20, 21].

The second exception is when an infection with *T. gondii* takes place in a pregnant woman. It has been known for many years that this can cause severe problems for the developing fetus, and for this reason, pregnant women are tested for toxoplasmosis infection by their obstetricians. If the infection takes place early in the pregnancy, the consequences may be especially severe, including spontaneous abortion, a stillborn child, or brain damage. Such damage may include an enlarged skull (hydrocephalus), calcifications of the brain tissue, or other brain damage producing seizures and/or decreased IQ, including mental retardation. It has been estimated that congenital toxoplasmosis infections occur in approximately 1 in 10,000 births in the United States, or approximately 3800 per year. Studies from France and Brazil that have provided a longer follow-up of possible cases have reported congenital infection rates up to ten times higher than the US study [22–24].

The third exception is that *T. gondii* is known to be a common cause of eye disease and, in fact, said to be "the most common retinal infection in the United States." Such infections occur commonly following congenital transmission, but they may also occur following infection in children and adults. For example, during the Canadian waterborne outbreak referred to above when 100 people became clinically symptomatic with toxoplasmosis, 20 of them had eye symptoms. Such symptoms may include eye pain, sensitivity to light, decreased vision, strabismus ("crossed eyes"), and nystagmus ("dancing eyes"), with severe cases even producing loss of vision. Either one or both eyes may be infected. It has been estimated that approximately 4800 individuals "develop symptomatic ocular toxoplasmosis each year in the United States" [25].

2.3   Fatal Attraction

Up until the turn of the twenty-first century, it was thought that the extent of human effects of *T. gondii* was confined to immunosuppressed individuals, congenital infections, and eye disease. Then in 2000 *T. gondii* was catapulted to public attention. In a highly publicized experiment, Joanne Webster and her colleagues at Oxford demonstrated that *T. gondii* was capable of altering the brains of rats, thus making it more likely that the *T. gondii*-infected rat would be eaten by a cat, thereby completing the life cycle of the parasite. It was, as the authors noted, a "fatal attraction." Specifically, rats were put in a room with cat urine in one corner and rabbit urine in another. Normal rats have a strong, hardwired aversion to cat urine, but the *T. gondii*-infected rats were actually attracted to it. This is an example of the manipulation hypothesis in evolutionary biology whereby "a parasite may alter the behavior of its host but for its own benefit, usually by enhancing its transmission rate." Another example is the malaria parasite which, when it infects humans, makes them more attractive to mosquitos which then further disseminate the parasite [26, 27].

The Oxford experiment caught the attention of the scientific community, resulting in headlines such as "How Your Cat is Making You Crazy" and "Can You Really Catch Madness from Your Cat?" Neuroscientist Robert Sapolsky and his colleagues at Stanford were among the first to replicate the study. They additionally demonstrated that the effect of the parasite on the rat brain was highly specific for only cat urine. The rat's reaction to the urine of other animals was not affected nor in general was its anxiety or fear altered. Sapolsky et al. claimed that "the behavioral syndrome produced by *T. gondii* does not have any precedent in neuroscience research." In a 2002 essay entitled "Bugs in the Brain," Sapolsky called the specificity of the brain manipulation by *T. gondii* "flabbergasting":

> This is akin to someone getting infected with a brain parasite that has no effect whatsoever on thoughts, emotions, SAT scores or television preferences but, to complete its life cycle, generates an irresistible urge to go to the zoo, scale a fence and try to French kiss the pissiest looking polar bear [28–30].

In the two decades since Webster et al. reported that rats infected with *T. gondii* had significant changes in their behavior, behavioral changes associated with *T.*

gondii have been reported in three other animal species. Wild red foxes exhibit facial muscle twitching, constant pacing, decreased fear of humans, and increased affection in what has been called the dopey fox syndrome. Hyena cubs that were infected with *T. gondii* were reported to have less fear of lions, as measured by their willingness to approach them, and to be 3.9 times more likely to be killed by them compared to cubs not infected. And chimpanzees, man's closest relatives, were shown to lose their innate aversion toward the urine of leopards, their only natural predator, when the chimpanzees become infected with *T. gondii* [31–34].

Such studies inevitably raised questions about the effects that *T. gondii* might be having on humans. Beginning in the 1990s, Jaroslav Flegr and his colleagues in Prague undertook a series of studies of personality characteristics comparing people who were, or were not, infected with *T. gondii*. They reported a variety of personality traits associated with this parasitic infection, which are more common in males and included being more "expedient, suspicious, jealous, and dogmatic." Such studies also have been carried out by other researchers, including in the United States; a 2018 summary of the studies claimed that the major personality characteristics of human *T. gondii* infection are greater impulsivity and aggressiveness. These studies raise the question of whether there are subgroups of Americans, among the 40 million so infected, who are unusually suspicious, impulsive, aggressive, etc. because they are infected with *T. gondii*. In one follow-up study, it was also reported that students who majored in business and people who start their own businesses were more likely than controls to be infected with *T. gondii*. Several recent studies have also suggested that toxoplasmosis may be responsible for causing mild cognitive impairment in some otherwise healthy people [35–39].

2.4   What Is the Evidence for Toxoplasmosis and Psychosis?

The 2000 publication by Webster et al. demonstrating that *T. gondii* can significantly change the behavior of animals was of great interest to those of us who had been researching infectious agents as a possible cause of schizophrenia and other psychoses. We were aware of reports that individuals infected with *T. gondii* occasionally had symptoms of psychosis. We were also aware of reports, beginning as early as 1953, that psychiatric patients often had increased antibodies to *T. gondii* compared to controls, indicating past infection. Almost all of these early studies had been carried out in Eastern Europe or China and were relatively unknown in Western Europe or America. In 1995 we published a paper asking "Could Schizophrenia Be a Viral Zoonosis Transmitted from House Cats?" [40].

The question was thus raised whether *Toxoplasma gondii* might be causing some cases of human psychosis, including people diagnosed with schizophrenia and bipolar disorder. Since it has been established that infectious agents in general can cause psychosis, as summarized in Chap. 1, it seemed like a reasonable question to ask. The following is the evidence supporting this possibility.

2.4.1 *T. gondii* Can Cause Psychotic Symptoms

It has been known for many years that *T. gondii* can cause delusions, auditory hallucinations, and other psychotic symptoms. As early as 1951, shortly after it had been first established that *T. gondii* could infect humans, a woman working with toxoplasmosis in a laboratory became infected, confirmed by a skin test. Among her symptoms were difficulties in concentrating or in following a conversation and feelings of being "far away, as if my body wasn't there." In 1966 a Dutch psychiatrist reported that "psychiatric disturbances were very frequent" in adults who acquired toxoplasmosis, occurring in 24 of 114 (21%) of the reviewed cases. Another Dutch researcher noted that "the literature not infrequently focuses attention on psychoses with schizophrenia or schizophreniform features that accompany chronic toxoplasmosis or that acquired in childhood or early in adult life." Among the cases was another laboratory worker who had become infected with *T. gondii* and then developed delusions and hallucinations. In more recent years, symptoms of psychosis have also frequently been seen in individuals with AIDS who develop a toxoplasmosis infection of the brain [41–43].

Relevant to the possible relationship between toxoplasmosis and psychosis is a clinical case on which I recently consulted. Two brothers, born 2 years apart, both developed schizophrenia in their teenage years. Although the mother had no known history of having had toxoplasmosis, the older brother had been diagnosed with toxoplasma eye disease at age 4. Since it is now known that congenital toxoplasmosis can be transmitted by an infected mother to more than one offspring, as noted above, this could theoretically produce multiple cases of psychosis in a family. If so, it would give schizophrenia or bipolar disorder the appearance of being a genetic disease when in fact it was really an infectious disease. In further support of such reasoning, eye symptoms, such as impaired visual acuity, nystagmus, and strabismus, are commonly found in individuals with schizophrenia as well as in toxoplasmosis eye disease. Retinal abnormalities are especially common in both schizophrenia and in toxoplasmosis eye disease [9, 44–48].

2.4.2 Among Individuals with Schizophrenia, Those Who Are Infected with *T. gondii* Have Been Shown to Have More Severe Symptoms

In one study, 57 individuals with schizophrenia who were infected with *T. gondii* were compared to 194 individuals with schizophrenia who were not infected. The infected group had more severe symptoms, were on higher doses of antipsychotic medications, and had been hospitalized longer. Another study of 94 individuals with schizophrenia reported a highly significant association between being infected with *T. gondii* and having a continuous and more severe course. In a third study, 210 inpatients, all of whom had had schizophrenia for at least 5 years, were divided into 100 who were characterized as treatment resistant and 110 who were not treatment resistant. Among the treatment resistant, 70% were found to be infected with *T.*

gondii compared to 36% of the nontreatment-resistant group. A study of 246 individuals with schizophrenia reported that those infected with toxoplasmosis were sicker, especially with more negative symptoms, than those not infected. A study of 600 individuals with first-episode schizophrenia reported significantly more delusions and hallucinations among those infected with *T. gondii.* Finally, a meta-analysis of 13 such studies concluded that "*T. gondii* infection has a modest effect on severity of positive and total symptoms in schizophrenia among those in the early stages of the disorder." It therefore appears that *T. gondii* infection is associated with a more severe form of schizophrenia [49–54].

2.4.3   Individuals with Psychosis, Compared to Controls, Are Significantly More Likely to Have Antibodies Against *T. gondii*, Indicating Past Infection

To date there have been approximately 100 such studies of individuals with schizophrenia, of which at least 80 have reported a significant association. For example, a 2012 meta-analysis of 38 studies, including 6067 individuals with schizophrenia and 8715 controls, reported an odds ratio of 2.7; in other words, a person who has been infected with *T. gondii* is 2.7 times more likely to have schizophrenia compared to a person who has not been infected. Similarly, a 2015 meta-analysis of 42 studies reported an odds ratio of 1.8. The single largest study, involving 81,962 blood donors in Denmark, reported a significant association between antibodies to *T. gondii* and a diagnosis of schizophrenia with an odds ratio of 1.5. When the data analysis was restricted to cases in which infection with *T. gondii* definitely preceded the onset of schizophrenia, the odds ratio was even higher: IRR 2.8 [55–57].

Similarly, there have been approximately 20 *T. gondii* antibody studies for individuals with bipolar disorder. One meta-analysis of 11 such studies reported a significant odds ratio of 1.5. A second meta-analysis of eight such studies, including five new ones, reported an odds ratio of 1.3. Most recently, the largest study done to date, involving 1207 bipolar patients and 745 controls, failed to find an association between *T. gondii* infection and bipolar disorder. Because only approximately one quarter of patients with bipolar disorder have psychotic symptoms, compared to all patients with schizophrenia, one would expect to find a weaker association [56, 58].

Other antibody studies have been carried out to ascertain whether a past infection with *T. gondii*, as assessed by having antibodies, can predict who is more likely to later develop psychosis. Five studies have assessed antibodies in women before they gave birth or in the newborn; four of the studies reported that the offspring of the women and the newborns who had antibodies to *T. gondii*, especially those with the highest titers, were significantly more likely to later develop schizophrenia or other psychoses. A recent review of these studies concluded: "The evidence provided by these newer studies strengthens the support for an association between prenatal exposure to *T. gondii* antibodies and risk of psychosis." An especially interesting study that used *T. gondii* antibodies to predict the later development of psychosis was carried out in China where 7126 entering university students were tested for

T. gondii antibody. By the end of 4 years, 84 students had developed psychosis. The entering students who had had evidence of past *T. gondii* infection (IgG antibodies) were 2.6 times more likely to develop psychosis; those who had evidence of a recent infection (IgM antibodies) were 5 times more likely to develop psychosis compared to the entering students who had not been infected by *T. gondii* [59–64].

2.4.4   Individuals with Schizophrenia or Bipolar Disorder, Compared to Controls, Are Significantly More Likely as a Child to Have Lived in a Home with a Cat

The first such study, published in 1995, included 165 individuals with schizophrenia or bipolar disorder and 165 matched controls. Those with schizophrenia or bipolar disorder were significantly more likely to have lived in a household with a cat, especially from ages 6 to 10. A follow-up study with 264 cases and 528 matched controls similarly reported a statistically significant excess of cat ownership between birth and age 13 among the individuals who later developed schizophrenia or bipolar disorder. A third study involving 2125 individuals with schizophrenia or bipolar disorder and 4847 controls reported a similar statistically significant difference—51% of the cases had owned a cat between birth and age 13 compared to 43% of the controls. All three of these studies were done in the United States using the membership of the National Alliance on Mental Illness (NAMI) [65–67].

There have been seven attempts to replicate these findings. In Turkey 300 hospitalized patients with schizophrenia were compared with 300 controls (150 blood donors and 150 nonpsychotic psychiatric outpatients) on family cat ownership in childhood, birth to age 13. Among those with schizophrenia, a statistically significant 59% had owned cats in childhood compared to 8% of the controls. In Tunisia, 200 individuals with serious mental illness were compared with 200 well-matched controls. Among the 101 patients diagnosed with schizophrenia, 59% had owned a cat during childhood compared to 38% of the controls, a statistically significant difference (Oumaima Inoubli, et al. "Childhood Cat Ownership is a Risk Factor for Schizophrenia at an Early Age," submitted for publication). In Canada, 1986 adults were asked about psychotic experiences and cat ownership prior to age 13. Those who reported having had psychotic experiences were significantly more likely to have owned a rodent-hunting (outside) cat in childhood than those who owned a non-rodent-hunting (inside) cat or no cat at all. In Finland cat ownership from birth up to the age of 7 was assessed in the northern Finland birth cohort. Cat ownership in early childhood was not significantly associated with the small number of 55 individuals diagnosed with schizophrenia but was significantly associated with the much larger group of 4866 individuals who were assessed for having schizotypal personality traits at age 31 [68–70].

In the Czech Republic, researchers collected online, self-reported data on Facebook from 8864 individuals regarding cat contact. Those who self-reported a diagnosis of bipolar disorder, but not schizophrenia, were significantly associated with having more cats in the house but not with cat ownership in childhood. In the

United States, a large cohort of 396 individuals with schizophrenia and 381 with bipolar disorder were compared to 594 controls on cat and dog ownership in childhood. Overall cat ownership was not a risk factor for either disease, but dog ownership was a significant protective factor against the development of schizophrenia. Finally, a study in England examined cat ownership at ages 4 and 10 in individuals who had some self-reported psychotic-like thinking at age 13. The initial association was statistically significant but was no longer significant when the researchers controlled for household crowding and poverty. Since household crowding and poverty have been clearly shown to increase the transmission of *T. gondii*, it may be argued that controlling for these factors is not appropriate and would weaken any association that did exist. In summary, among ten studies of cat ownership in childhood and the later development of psychotic symptoms, six studies reported a significant association, two reported mixed results, and two studies were negative [71–74].

In fact it is surprising that it is possible in any study to find a significant association between cat ownership in childhood and psychosis. Children can become infected in many different locations that are contaminated with *T. gondii* oocysts, including play areas at school, a babysitter's house, a friend's house, or a public park. Even if a child became infected in a sandbox at their own home, they would not necessarily have to have owned a cat; cats from the neighborhood may well be responsible for the oocyst contamination.

2.5   How Many Cases of Psychosis Might Be Caused by *T. gondii*?

Overall, the evidence suggests that *T. gondii* might cause some cases of psychosis. Is there any way to estimate how many cases this might be? In 2014, Dr. Gary Smith in the School of Veterinary Medicine at the University of Pennsylvania published a paper in which he tried to answer this question specifically for schizophrenia. Using data from the *T. gondii* antibody studies discussed above, he estimated the population attributable fraction of cases of schizophrenia that were likely to be caused by the parasite to 21% with a possible range from 14% to 31%. Regarding the annual incidence of schizophrenia, the most recent international data suggests that it is approximately 14.6 cases per hundred thousand population. Based on the US population of 330 million, that rate would translate into 48,100 new cases of schizophrenia each year. And 21% of that would be approximately 10,300 cases attributable to *T. gondii* [75, 76].

Nobody has yet done a similar study to calculate the population attributable fraction of cases of affective psychosis, which would include bipolar disorder and severe depression with psychotic features, but let us assume that it is also 21%. The annual incidence of affective psychosis is 7.1 per hundred thousand population. That rate translates into approximately 23,400 new cases of affective psychosis each year, of which 4900 would be attributable to *T. gondii*. Altogether, then, the protozoal parasite that causes toxoplasmosis might be responsible for approximately 15,000 new cases of psychosis in the United States each year.

In fact, estimating the population attributable fraction of cases of psychosis that may be caused by *T. gondii* is very difficult because there are so many unknowns. Some of these unknowns include the following:

- *Inaccurate testing*: It has become increasingly clear that the tests being used to ascertain whether or not a person has been infected with *T. gondii* are often not accurate. This is especially true for individuals, such as those with schizophrenia or bipolar disorder, who are taking antipsychotic medications which are thought to suppress the immune response. This was demonstrated most clearly in a study in which 39 individuals with schizophrenia who had never been treated and 36 individuals with schizophrenia who were being treated were compared with 73 normal controls. On *T. gondii* antibody testing, of both the serum and cerebrospinal fluid, the patients who had never been treated had statistically significant higher antibody levels then the controls. The patients who were being treated had lower antibody levels than those who were not being treated, slightly but not significantly higher than normal controls. This suggests that for individuals receiving antipsychotic medication, many are being classified falsely as not being infected with *T. gondii*. This is also true for individuals being immunosuppressed; for example, in a study of AIDS patients, 16% of those known to be infected with *T. gondii* tested negative for antibodies. Other studies have shown that antibodies to *T. gondii* may wane over time even in individuals with live cysts in the brain. Of special concern was a recent study in mice in which male mice whose sperm was infected with *T. gondii* altered the behavior of their offspring through RNA changes, even though the offspring themselves had no antibodies to toxoplasmosis. Whether or not this also happens in humans is not known [77–81].
- *Host genetics*: For most infectious agents, it is known that some people are genetically more susceptible to becoming infected, while others are genetically more resistant. This is also true for *T. gondii*. For example, it has been shown that if an individual has a particular gene (HLA-DQ3), that person will be more susceptible to getting toxoplasmosis that affects the brain. On the other hand, if a person has a different gene (HLA-DQ1), that person will be more resistant to such infections [82].
- *Immune status*: The effectiveness of a person's immune system in fighting off assaults by infectious agents varies widely among individuals and also in a given individual over time. Thus if you also have the flu when you are exposed to *T. gondii*, your immune system may be weakened. This principle has been demonstrated by individuals with AIDS who have impaired immune systems and in whom *T. gondii* often causes major brain infections.
- *Form of infectious agent*: *T. gondii* may infect people as an oocyst (e.g., in contaminated water) or as a tissue cyst (for example, in undercooked lamb). In mice

it has been shown that infections with oocysts lead to more severe disease than infections with tissue cysts. Similarly, according to one toxoplasmosis expert, "circumstantial evidence suggests that oocyst-induced infections in humans are clinically more severe than tissue cyst-acquired infections" [83].

- *Strain*: *T. gondii* is known to have many strains, some being much more pathogenic than others. Type I, II, and III strains have been most widely studied, but almost 200 other genotypes have been identified. Different strains are known to have markedly different effects on animals; for example, type I kills mice, but types II and III do not. In humans, type I is thought to cause most cases of congenital toxoplasmosis as well as eye disease. In an important study of 91 women who had had toxoplasmosis and gave birth to individuals who developed psychosis, an association was statistically significant for women who had been infected with a type I strain, but not for those infected with type II or III strains. It has also been shown in humans that different strains affect brain neurotransmitters and neuropeptides very differently, so it would be expected that different strains would have different psychiatric effects. Sorting this out is made more difficult by the fact that a person may become infected with more than one strain [63, 84–88].

- *Timing of infection*: For many infectious agents, it is known that the specific timing of the infection in human development is a major determinant in the outcome. For example, the polio virus may have a very different effect if it infects a 2-year-old rather than a 12-year-old. Timing is also thought to be important for *T. gondii*. Studies in mice reported very different outcomes, including the effects on neurotransmitters, when mice were infected as juveniles or as adults. The importance of timing is also suggested by congenital toxoplasmosis; the outcome of first trimester infections is much worse than the outcome of third trimester infections [89].

- *Breed of cat*: The susceptibility of cats to infection by *T. gondii* varies significantly by breed. A study carried out in Finland on 1121 cats representing 8 different breeds reported a threefold difference in Toxoplasma seropositivity. The cats with the highest rate of infection were Persians at 60%, and those with the lowest rate were Burmese at 19%; the other 6 breeds had intermediate rates. In general the longhaired breeds were twice as likely to be infected as the shorthaired breeds. Since cat breeds tend to be regionally popular and to change over time, this would be another variable that would affect the prevalence of toxoplasmosis. Thus two countries could have the same number of cats, but, because they favor different breeds, one country could have twice as much toxoplasmosis as the other [90].

In summary, there is still much we do not understand regarding human infections with *T. gondii*. This parasite has provided many surprises so far and is likely to provide still more.

2.6   Other Diseases and Conditions

As interest in *Toxoplasma gondii* has increased in the last two decades, researchers have looked for associations of this parasite with other diseases and conditions. Given the propensity of *T. gondii* to infect the brain and the reports of its association with psychosis, researchers have looked especially at diseases and conditions associated with the brain. These have included autism, Alzheimer's disease, Parkinson's disease, multiple sclerosis, cerebral palsy, and suicidal behavior. Among the studies the diseases and conditions that show the strongest associations with *T. gondii* are epilepsy, brain cancer, rheumatoid arthritis, and motor vehicle accidents.

Epilepsy   Since 1995, 16 studies have been published looking for an association between toxoplasmosis and epilepsy. A 2015 meta-analysis of 6 of these studies, with a total of 1280 subjects with epilepsy and 1608 controls, reported a positive association with an odds ratio of 2.25, $p = 0.005$. The authors concluded that "despite the limited number of studies and lack of high-quality data, toxoplasmosis should continue to be regarded as an epilepsy risk factor." A recent meta-analysis that included all 16 studies, with 3771 epileptic patients and 4026 healthy controls, reported an odds ratio of 1.72, $p = 0.001$ [91, 92].

Brain cancer   Since 1967 there have been five case-control and two epidemiological published studies on the relationship between infection with *T. gondii* and brain cancer. A study in Minnesota of 24 meningiomas, tumors of the covering of the brain, and 77 gliomas, tumors of the brain substance, reported that both were increased in individuals infected with *T. gondii*, but this only achieved statistical significance for the 35 gliomas categorized as astrocytomas ($p < 0.01$). A study in Australia looked for infection in 53 individuals with meningiomas and 117 with gliomas. The former showed a significant association ($p < 0.02$; OR 2.09), but the latter showed no increase. A Korean study examined 93 brain cancers, including 12 meningiomas, 14 astrocytomas, and 31 glioblastomas; all 3 were significantly associated with *T. gondii* infection at the $p < 0.05$ level. Most recently two prospective studies were published, meaning that the blood was collected to ascertain *T. gondii* status before the brain tumor was diagnosed. A small study of 37 gliomas from the United States and a large study of 328 gliomas from Norway both reported a significant association with toxoplasmosis infection (OR 2.70 and OR 1.32 respectively). In summary, two out of the three studies of meningiomas and four out of the five studies of gliomas reported a statistically significant association between the brain cancer and infection with *T. gondii* [93–96].

   The first of the two epidemiological studies was published in 2012 and involved data from 37 countries. The national incidence of brain cancers was compared to the national rate of *T. gondii* seropositivity. The authors reported a significant association, specifically "infection with *T. gondii* was associated with a 1.8-fold increase in the risk of brain cancers." The authors attempted to replicate these findings by comparing similar data for the 22 administrative regions of France. They reported a similar significant association but only for men age 55 and over and women age 65 and over with the magnitude of the effect increasing with age [97, 98].

Rheumatoid arthritis   Perhaps the most interesting association of *T. gondii* with other diseases is with rheumatoid arthritis. Eight studies have reported an increased prevalence of *T. gondii* antibodies in individuals with this disease. A meta-analysis of these studies, with 1244 patients and 2799 controls, reported an odds ratio of 3.30, $p < 0.0001$. Another study reported that individuals with rheumatoid arthritis, compared to controls, have had more exposure to cats. This association is especially interesting because rheumatoid arthritis and schizophrenia share several epidemiological features, and it has been noted in many studies that the two diseases are mutually exclusive, i.e., once you get either rheumatoid arthritis or schizophrenia, you almost never get the other. This suggests that *T. gondii* or another pathogen may cause some cases of both diseases with the clinical outcome differing because of genetic predisposition, timing of the initial infection, strain difference, or other factor [99, 100].

Motor vehicle accidents   Laboratory work with mice infected with *T. gondii* established the fact that the parasite causes a slowing of their reaction time. Therefore in 2001 Jaroslav Flegr and his colleagues in Prague compared the reaction time of 60 human subjects infected with the parasite and 56 subjects not infected. Those infected had a significantly longer reaction time. Based on these findings, Flegr et al. wondered whether this might have practical implications, such as increasing the rate of vehicular accidents in individuals who were infected [101].

Flegr et al. compared 146 drivers who had caused an accident and pedestrians who had been hit by a vehicle with 446 local residents. The drivers and pedestrians were significantly more likely to be infected with *T. gondii* with an odds ratio of 2.65 ($p < 0.0001$). Since that study was published, ten other studies have been done in Denmark, Poland, Russia, Czech Republic, Turkey, Mexico, and New Zealand, half reporting positive results and half reporting negative results. The largest of these was the Danish study involving 2724 drivers in accidents and 6294 matched control blood donors and reported "a very weak association between traffic accidents and toxoplasmosis" (OR 1.11; $p = 0.054$). A meta-analysis done on all the studies reported an odds ratio of 1.69 ($p = 0.003$) [102–104].

Such data should always be approached with caution, however, since correlations do not necessarily indicate causation. As one observer noted, "Think of people who enjoy rare steaks and also tend to drive recklessly in fast cars. Consuming rare meat raises their chances of [toxoplasmosis] infection and reckless driving makes their chances of an accident more likely, but personal taste could explain the link between infections and accidents rather than parasite control" [105].

In summary, Chap. 1 established the fact that many human diseases are transmitted to us by infectious agents from animals as well as the fact that infectious agents can cause psychosis. Chapter 2 has proposed that *Toxoplasma gondii*, a protozoan parasite carried by cats, may cause some cases of psychosis, specifically schizophrenia and bipolar disorder. Is there additional evidence that might support such a claim? Historically cats have a very unusual and distinctive history. For 400 years they were used for rodent control but kept in the barn, socially shunned as agents of Satan and on religious holidays tortured and killed. Then over the next 400 years, they slowly became pets for humans, then companions and finally family members. The relationship between cats and humans, and thus human exposure to *Toxoplasma gondii*, changed radically over the eight centuries. If there really is a relationship between this parasite and human psychosis, wouldn't we expect to see some correlation between the changing relationship between cats and humans and the incidence of psychosis?

Among English-speaking nations, there is only one country which has sufficient data to address this question. England has extensive anecdotal data on the status of cats because its writers embraced them as pets and wrote about them. It also has extensive information on the incidence and prevalence of psychosis, usually referred to as madness or insanity. It is thus to England that we now turn for the next three chapters to ascertain whether there is any correlation between the rise of cats and the rise of madness.

References

1. Joynson DHM, Wreghitt TG, editors. Toxoplasmosis: a comprehensive clinical guide. New York: Cambridge University Press; 2001. p. xi.
2. Harker KS, et al. *Toxoplasma gondii* dissemination: a parasite's journey through the infected host. Parasite Immunol. 2015;37(3):141–9. https://doi.org/10.1111/pim.12163.
3. Jones JL, et al. *Toxoplasma gondii* infestation in the United States, 2011–2014. Am J Trop Med Hyg. 2018;98:551–7.
4. Ben-Harari RR. High burden and low awareness of Toxoplasma in the United States. Postgrad Med. 2019;131:103–8.
5. Kodjikian L, et al. Vertical transmission of toxoplasmosis from a chronically infected immunocompetent woman. Pediatr Infect Dis J. 2004;23(3):272–4. https://doi.org/10.1097/01. inf.0000115949.12206.69.
6. Lass A, et al. The first detection of *Toxoplasma gondii* DNA in environmental air samples using gelatine filters, real-time PCR and loop-mediated isothermal (LAMP) assays. Parasitology. 2017;144:1791–801.
7. Teutsch SM, et al. Epidemic toxoplasmosis associated with infected cats. N Engl J Med. 1979;300:695–9.
8. Stagno S, et al. An outbreak of toxoplasmosis linked to cats. Pediatrics. 1980;65:706–12.
9. Asbell PA, et al. Presumed toxoplasmic retinochoroiditis in four siblings. Am J Ophthalmol. 1982;94(5):656–63.
10. Kean BH, et al. An epidemic of acute toxoplasmosis. JAMA. 1969;208:1002–4.
11. Jones JL, Dubey JP. Foodborne toxoplasmosis. Clin Infect Dis. 2012;55:845–51.
12. Dubey JP. Toxoplasmosis—a waterborne zoonosis. Clin Infect Dis. 2012;55:845–51.
13. Dubey JP. Outbreaks of clinical toxoplasmosis in humans: five decades of personal experience, perspectives, and lessons learned. Parasite Vectors. 2021;14:263–75.
14. Bowie WR, et al. Outbreak of toxoplasmosis associated with municipal drinking water. Lancet. 1997;350:173–7.
15. Bik HM, et al. Microbial community patterns associated with automated teller machine keypads in New York City. msphere. 2016;1:e00223-16. https://doi.org/10.1128/mSphere.0026-16.
16. Pawełczyk O, et al. The discovery of zoonotic protozoans in fleas parasitizing on pets as a potential infection threat. Acta Parasitol. 2020;65(4):817–22. https://doi.org/10.2478/s11686-020-00221-2.
17. Arantes TP, et al. *Toxoplasma gondii*: evidence for the transmission by semen in dogs. Exp Parasitol. 2009;123:190–4.

18. Lopes WDZ, et al. Sexual transmission of *Toxoplasma gondii* in sheep. Vet Parasitol. 2013;195:47–56.
19. Disko R, et al. Untersucheungen zum Vorkommen von *Toxoplasma gondii* im menschlichen Ejakulat. Z Tropenmed Parasitol. 1971;22:391–6.
20. Belk K, et al. Patient and treatment pathways for toxoplasmosis in the United States: data analysis of the Vizient Health Systems data from 2011 to 2017. Pathog Glob Health. 2018;112(8):428–37. https://doi.org/10.1080/20477724.2018.1552644.
21. Cummings PL, et al. Trends, productivity losses, and associated medical conditions among toxoplasmosis deaths in the United States, 2000–2010. Am J Trop Med Hyg. 2014;91(5):959–64. https://doi.org/10.4269/ajtmh.14-0287.
22. Kalantari N, et al. *Toxoplasma gondii* infection in spontaneous abortion: a systematic review and metanalysis. Microb Pathog. 2021;158:105070. https://doi.org/10.1016/j.micpath.2021.105070.
23. Guerina NG, et al. Neonatal serologic screening and early treatment for congenital *Toxoplasma gondii* infection. The New England Regional Toxoplasma Working Group. N Engl J Med. 1994;330(26):1858–63. https://doi.org/10.1056/NEJM199406303302604.
24. Dubey JP, et al. Congenital toxoplasmosis in humans: an update of worldwide rate of infections. Parasitology. 2021. https://doi.org/10.1017/S0031182021001013.
25. Jones JL, Holland GN. Annual burden of ocular toxoplasmosis in the US. Am J Trop Med Hyg. 2010;82:464–5. https://doi.org/10.4269/ajtmh.2010.09-0664.
26. Berdoy M, et al. Fatal attraction in rats infected with *toxoplasma gondii*. Proc R Soc Lond. 2000;267:1591–4.
27. Lacroix R, et al. Malaria infection increases attractiveness of humans to mosquitos. PLoS Biol. 2005;3:1590–3.
28. Vyas A, et al. Behavioral changes induced by *Toxoplasma* infection of rodents are highly specific to aversion of cat odors. PNAS. 2007;104:6442–7.
29. Vyas A, Sapolsky R. Manipulation of host behavior by *Toxoplasma gondii*. Folia Parasitol. 2010;57:88–94.
30. Sapolsky R. Bugs in the brain. Sci Am. 2003:94–7.
31. Milne G, et al. Infectious causation of abnormal host behavior: *Toxoplasma gondii* and its potential association with Dopey Fox syndrome. Front Psychiatry. 2020;11:513536. https://doi.org/10.3389/fpsyt.2020.513536.
32. Miller MA, et al. An unusual genotype of *Toxoplasma gondii* is common in California sea otters (Enhydra lutris nereis) and is a cause of mortality. Int J Parasitol. 2004;34(3):275–84. https://doi.org/10.1016/j.ijpara.2003.12.008.
33. Gering E, et al. *Toxoplasma gondii* infections are associated with costly boldness towards felids in a wild host. Nat Commun. 2021;12:3842. https://doi.org/10.1038/s41467-021-24092-x.
34. Poirotte C, et al. Morbid attraction to leopard urine in toxoplasma-infected chimpanzees. Curr Biol. 2016;26(3):R98–9. https://doi.org/10.1016/j.cub.2015.12.020.
35. Flegr J. Effects of toxoplasma on human behavior. Schizophr Bull. 2007;33(3):757–60. https://doi.org/10.1093/schbul/sbl074.
36. Martinez VO, et al. *Toxoplasma gondii* infection and behavioral outcomes in humans: a systematic review. Parasitol Res. 2018;117(10):3059–65. https://doi.org/10.1007/s00436-018-6040-2.
37. Coccaro EF. *Toxoplasma gondii* infection: relationship with aggression in psychiatric subjects. J Clin Psychiatry. 2016;77:334–41.
38. Johnson SK, et al. Risky business: linking *Toxoplasma gondii* infection and entrepreneurship behaviours across individuals and countries. Proc Biol Sci. 2018;285(1883):20180822. https://doi.org/10.1098/rspb.2018.0822.
39. Lies de Haan, et al. Association of *Toxoplasma gondii* seropositivity with cognitive function in healthy people: a systematic review and meta-analysis. JAMA Psychiatry. https://doi.org/10.1001/jamapsychiatry.2021.1590.
40. Torrey EF and Yolken RH. Could schizophrenia be a viral zoonosis transmitted from house cats? Schizophr Bull. 1995;21(2):167–71.

41. Strom J. Toxoplasmosis due to laboratory infestation in two adults. Acta Med Scand. 1951;139:244–52.
42. Kramer W. Frontiers of neurological diagnosis in acquired toxoplasmosis. Psychiatr Neurol Neurochir. 1966;69:43–54.
43. Ladee GA, et al. Diagnostic problems in psychiatry with regard to acquired toxoplasmosis. Psychiatr Neurol Neurochir. 1966;69:65–82.
44. Ladas ID, et al. Presumed congenital ocular toxoplasmosis in two successive siblings. Ophthalmologica. 1999;213(5):320–2.
45. Lou P, et al. Ocular toxoplasmosis in three consecutive siblings. Arch Ophthalmol. 1978;96(4):613–4.
46. Torrey EF, Yolken RH. Schizophrenia and infections: the eyes have it. Schizophr Bull. 2017;43(2):247–52.
47. Adams S, Nasrallah H. Multiple retinal anomalies in schizophrenia. Schizophr Res. 2018;195:3–12.
48. Appaji A, et al. Retinal vascular tortuosity in schizophrenia and bipolar disorder. Schizophr Res. 2019;212:26–32.
49. Holub D, et al. Differences in onset of disease and severity of psychopathology between toxoplasmosis-related and toxoplasmosis-unrelated schizophrenia. Acta Psychiatr Scand. 2013;127:227–38.
50. Celik T, et al. Association between latent toxoplasmosis and clinical course of schizophrenia—continuous course of the disease is characteristic for *Toxoplasma gondii*-infected patients. Folia Parasitol. 2015;62:2015.015.
51. Vlatkovic S, et al. Increased prevalence of *Toxoplasma gondii* seropositivity in patients with treatment-resistant schizophrenia. Schizophr Res. 2018;193:480–1.
52. Esshili A, et al. *Toxoplasma gondii* infection in schizophrenia and associated clinical features. Psychiatry Res. 2016;245:327–32.
53. Wang H-L, et al. Prevalence of *Toxoplasma* infection in first episode schizophrenia and comparison between *Toxoplasma*-seropositive and *Toxoplasma*-negative schizophrenia. Acta Psychiatr Scand. 2006;120:40–8.
54. Sutterland A, et al. *Toxoplasma gondii* infection and clinical characteristics of patients with schizophrenia: a systematic review and meta-analysis. Poster, Schizophrenia International Research Society meeting, April 17–20, 2021.
55. Torrey EF, et al. *Toxoplasma gondii* and other risk factors for schizophrenia: an update. Schizophr Bull. 2012;38:642–7.
56. Sutterland AL, et al. Beyond the association: *Toxoplasma gondii* in schizophrenia, bipolar disorder and addiction: systematic review and meta-analysis. Acta Psychiatr Scand. 2015;132:161–79.
57. Burgdorf KS, et al. Large-scale serology study of toxoplasma and cytomegalovirus in relation to psychiatric disorders, suicide behaviors and risk of traffic accidents. Brain Behav Immun. 2019;79:152–8.
58. Frye MA, et al. Association of cytomegalovirus and *Toxoplasma gondii* antibody titers with bipolar disorder. JAMA Psychiat. 2019;76(12):1285–93.
59. Mortensen PB, et al. *Toxoplasma gondii* as a risk factor for early-onset schizophrenia: analysis of filter paper blood sample obtained as birth. Biol Psychiatry. 2007;61:688–92.
60. Blomstrom A, et al. Maternal antibodies to infectious agents and risk for non-affective psychoses in the offspring: a matched case-control study. Schizophr Res. 2012;140:25–30.
61. Brown AS, et al. Maternal exposure to toxoplasmosis and risk of schizophrenia in adult offspring. Am J Psychiatr. 2005;162:767–73.
62. Buka SL, et al. Maternal infections and subsequent psychosis among offspring. Arch Gen Psychiatry. 2001;58:1032–7.
63. Xiao J, et al. Serological infection consistent with type I *Toxoplasma gondii* in mothers and risk of psychosis among adult offspring. Microb Infect. 2007;11:1011–8.
64. Cheslack-Postava K, Brown AS. Prenatal infection and schizophrenia: a decade of further progress. Schizophr Res. 2021. https://doi.org/10.1016/j.schres.2021.05.014.

65. Torrey EF and Yolken RH. Could schizophrenia be a viral zoonoses transmitted from house cats? Schizophr Bull. 1995;21:167–71.
66. Torrey EF, et al. The antecedents of psychosis: a case-control study of selected risk factors. Schizophr Res. 2000;46:17–23.
67. Torrey EF, et al. Is childhood cat ownership a risk factor for schizophrenia later in life? Schizophr Res. 2015;165:1–2.
68. Yuksel P, et al. The role of latent toxoplasmosis in the aetiopathogenesis of schizophrenia—the risk factor or an indication of a contact with cat? Folia Parasitol. 2010;57:121–8.
69. Paquin V, et al. Cat ownership in childhood has sex-specific associations with psychotic experiences and interacts with other risk-factors in a community sample. Poster, Schizophrenia International Research Society meeting, April 17–20, 2021.
70. Palomaki J, et al. Cat ownership in childhood and development of schizophrenia. Lett Schizophr Res. 2019;206:444–5.
71. Flegr J, Vedralova M. Specificity and nature of the association of twenty-four neuropsychiatric disorders with contacts with cats and dogs. Lett Schizophr Res. 2017;189:219–20.
72. Yolken RH, et al. Exposure to household pet cats and dogs in childhood and risk of subsequent diagnosis of schizophrenia. PLoS One. 2019;14(12):e0225320.
73. Solmi F, et al. Curiosity killed the cat: no evidence of an association between cat ownership and psychotic symptoms of ages 13 and 18 in a UK general population cohort. Psychol Med. 2017;22:1–9.
74. Torrey EF, Yolken RH. How statistics killed the cat. Lett Psychol Med. 2018;48:175.
75. Smith G. Estimating the population attributable fraction for schizophrenia when *Toxoplasma gondii* is assumed absent in human populations. Prev Vet Med. 2014;117(3–4):425–35.
76. Castillejos MC, et al. A systematic review and meta-analysis of the incidence of psychotic disorders: the distribution of rates and the influence of gender, urbanicity, immigration and socioeconomic level. Psychol Med. 2018:1–15. https://doi.org/10.1017/S0033291718000235.
77. Leweke MF, et al. Antibodies for infectious agents in individuals with recent onset schizophrenia. Eur Arch Psychiatry Clin Neurosci. 2004;254:4–8.
78. Porter S, Sande M. Toxoplasmosis of the central nervous system in the acquired immunodeficiency syndrome. N Engl J Med. 1992;327(23):1643–8. https://doi.org/10.1056/NEJM199212033272306.
79. Van Durten H, et al. Epidemiologic implications of limited-duration seropositivity after toxoplasma infection. Am J Epidemiol. 1990;32:169–80.
80. Konishi E. Annual change in immunoglobulin G and M antibody levels to *Toxoplasma gondii* in human sera. Microbiol Immunol. 1989;33(5):403–11.
81. Tyebji S, et al. Pathogenic infection in male mice changes sperm small RNA profiles and transgenerationally alters offspring behavior. Cell Rep. 2020;31(4):107573.
82. Suzuki Y. Host resistance in the brain against *Toxoplasma gondii*. J Infect Dis. 2002;185(Suppl 1):558–65.
83. Dubey JP. Toxoplasmosis-a waterborne zoonosis. Vet Parasitol. 2004;126:57–72.
84. Xiao J, Yolken RH. Strain hypothesis of *Toxoplasma gondii* infection on the outcome of human disease. Acta Physiol. 2015;213:828–45.
85. Xia J, et al. Association between *Toxoplasma gondii* types and outcomes of human infection: a meta-analysis. Acta Microbiol Immunol Hung. 2017;64:1–16.
86. Rico-Torres CP, et al. Is *Toxoplasma gondii* type related to clinical outcome in human congenital infection? Eur J Clin Microbiol Infect Dis. 2016;35:1079–88.
87. Shobab L, et al. Toxoplasma serotype is associated with development of ocular toxoplasmosis. J Infect Dis. 2013;208:1520–8.
88. Xiao J, et al. Abnormalities of neurotransmitter and neuropeptide systems in human neuroepithelioma cells infected by three toxoplasma strains. J Neural Transm. 2013;120:1631–9.
89. Kannan G, et al. Anti-NMDA receptor autoantibodies and associated neurobehavioral pathology in mice are dependent on age of first exposure to *Toxoplasma gondii*. Neurobiol Dis. 2016;91:307–14.

90. Must K, et al. *Toxoplasma gondii* seroprevalence varies by cat breed. PloS One. 2017;12(9):e0184659. https://doi.org/10.1371/journal.pone.0184659.
91. Ngoungou EB, et al. Toxoplasmosis and epilepsy: systemic review and meta-analysis. PLoS Negl Trop Dis. 2015;9:e0003525.
92. Sadeghi M, et al. An updated meta-analysis of the association between *Toxoplasma gondii* infection and risk of epilepsy. Trans R Soc Trop Med Hyg. 2019;113(8):453–62.
93. Schuman LM, et al. Relationship of central nervous system neoplasms to *Toxoplasma gondii* infection. Am J Public Health Nations Health. 1967;57(5):848–56.
94. Ryan P, et al. Tumours of the brain and presence of antibodies to *Toxoplasma gondii*. Int J Epidemiol. 1993;22:412–9.
95. Jung B-K, et al. High *Toxoplasma gondii* seropositivity among brain tumor patients in Korea. Korean J Parasitol. 2016;54:201–4.
96. Hodge JM, et al. *Toxoplasma gondii* infection and the risk of adult glioma in two prospective studies. Int J Cancer. 2021;148:2449–56.
97. Thomas F, et al. Incidence of adult brain cancers is higher in countries where the protozoan parasite *Toxoplasma gondii* is common. Biol Lett. 2012;8(1):101–3.
98. Vittecoq M, et al. Brain cancer mortality rates increase with *Toxoplasma gondii* seroprevalence in France. Infect Genet Evol. 2012;12:496–8.
99. Hosseininejad Z, et al. Toxoplasmosis seroprevalence in rheumatoid arthritis patients: a systematic review and meta-analysis. PLoS Negl Trop Dis. 2018;12:e0006545.
100. Gottlieb NL, et al. Pets and rheumatoid arthritis: an epidemiological survey. Arthritis Rheum. 1974;17:229–34.
101. Havlícek J, et al. Decrease of psychomotor performance in subjects with latent 'asymptomatic' toxoplasmosis. Parasitology. 2001;122:515–20.
102. Flegr J, et al. Increased risk of traffic accidents in subjects with latent toxoplasmosis: a retrospective case-control study. BMC Infect Dis. 2002;2. https://doi.org/10.1186/1471-2334-2-11.
103. Burgdorf KS, et al. Large-scale study of toxoplasma and cytomegalovirus shows an association between infection and serious psychiatric disorders. Brain Behav Immun. 2019;79:152–8.
104. Sutterland AL, et al. Driving us mad: the association of *Toxoplasma gondii* with suicide attempts and traffic accidents – a systematic review and meta-analysis. Psychol Med. 2019;49(10):1608–23.
105. Wood C. www.brainfacts.org. Feline parasites influence rat behavior but what about cat lovers? June 12, 2020. https://www.brainfacts.org/in-the-lab/animals-in-research/2020/feline-parasites-influence-rat-behavior-but-what-about-cat-lovers-061120.

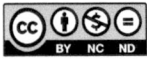

The Rise of Cats and Madness: I. The Renaissance

3

3.1 Cats and Satan

From the middle of the thirteenth century until the end of the Renaissance, cats were regarded as utilitarian creatures to guard food supplies from rodents. Otherwise, except for a small group of artists, writers, and clerics, most people regarded cats as being associated with the Devil. During these years madness was relatively uncommon and, in most cases, caused by medical conditions which had existed for many centuries.

To understand the profound change that has occurred in our relationship with cats over the past five centuries, one must first understand how they developed such a bad reputation. Their road to infamy began in 30 BCE when Roman forces under Octavian defeated Egypt and made it a Roman province. The Romans then imported the Egyptian goddess Isis and her companion, the cat-headed goddess, Bastet. According to Donald Engels' book on *Classical Cats*, "The enormous popularity of Isis during the Roman Empire cannot be stressed enough: there are vast quantities of dedicatory inscriptions, votive offerings, altars and temples dedicated to her throughout Europe." Over time Isis merged with the Roman goddess Diana, the goddess of the hunt and nature. As her companion, Bastet protected women and children and was also associated with fertility and childbirth. The Isis-Diana-Bastet religious cult was especially popular with women and spread throughout Southern Europe as the Roman Empire extended its reach. Thus the cat became an important symbol for a religion that became increasingly widespread [1].

At the same time as Roman administrators and traders were disseminating a cat-related religion across Europe, the Roman army was disseminating cats. Cats were important to the army to protect its food supplies and were also regarded as symbols of good luck. According to one source, "a cat was often emblazoned on the shields and flags of Roman soldiers." Thus, for example, cats were brought to England by Roman legions who invaded in 43 CE under Emperor Claudius. After defeating the Celts, Claudius entered their capital at Colchester "at the head of an army made

© E. Fuller Torrey 2022
E. F. Torrey, *Parasites, Pussycats and Psychosis*,
https://doi.org/10.1007/978-3-030-86811-6_3

doubly impressive by elephants." The Romans would remain in England for almost 400 years [2, 3].

Although the cult of Diana was widespread in Southern Europe, other religions existed in the north. There the various tribes of Teutonic stock, including the Goths, Franks, Saxons, Angeles, and Jutes, had largely resisted the Romans and their influence. Many of them followed the Norse religion and worshipped Odin, also known as Wotan, the warrior god; his son Thor (the origin of Thursday), the thunder god; and Freya (the origin of Friday) the fertility goddess and sister-in-law of Odin. The importance of these deities was illustrated by the description of a Norse temple in Uppsala, Sweden:

> In the great temple, 900 ells [450 yards] in circumference, and glittering on all sides with gold, stood the image of Odin, sword in hand. In his right was Freya, with the emblem of fertility, and on his left Thor with his hammer.

All of these deities play roles in Richard Wagner's four nineteenth-century operas, "Der Ring des Nibelungen" [4].

Freya, like Isis and Diana, was strongly associated with cats, two of which were said to pull the chariot by which she traveled. According to one source, "the warriors in the ancient German tribes, unacquainted with big cats [such as lions], made the European wildcat an emblem of courage," and thus it is not surprising that cats have an important place in their religion. Pictures of Freya with two cats have been found dated to as early as the seventh century, so the association was very old. In addition to fertility, Freya was associated with love, sex, war, and death, and she presided over the afterlife of half the warriors who died in battle; the other half went to Odin's hall, Valhalla [5].

Prior to the reign of the Roman Emperor Constantine (306–337 CE), Christianity was one of many religious sects in Rome, and its adherents were frequently persecuted. In 313 CE, Constantine issued an edict prohibiting further persecution and became a Christian himself. In 380 CE Christianity was made the official religion of the Roman Empire.

Thus began a struggle that would last for a thousand years to establish Christianity throughout Europe and beyond. The struggle involved internal divisions of Christianity, such as the Cathars and Waldensians who had their own ideas regarding how Christianity should be practiced and challenged the church's orthodoxy. The struggle also involved external challenges to convert the "pagans" who worshipped deities such as Isis, Diana, and Freya.

Many of the existing religions did not meekly accept Christianity. For example, in the sixth century, after the fall of the Roman Empire, Saxons from Northern Germany invaded Britain and "showed a special hatred of Christianity. They destroyed the churches…slew the clergy, burnt the sacred books, and did their utmost to extinguish the faith." Attempts by Christians to convert groups such as the Saxons were equally brutal, often based on a choice between being converted or being killed. For example, in 782 CE, Charlemagne, who was the Christian king of the Franks, defeated the Saxons at Verden in Northern Germany and ordered all 4500 captives to be beheaded in a single day [6].

Despite such tactics, many northerners were reluctant to abandon their traditional gods. It has been claimed that "a majority of the French peasantry, and hence the French people, were still practicing pagans through the eleventh century and even beyond…Female divinities were especially popular among women… A statue of Isis continued to be worshipped in the church of St. Germain-des-Pres in Paris through the thirteenth century, before it was finally removed and smashed." The worship of Bastet survived in Ypres, Belgium, "through AD 962 when the cult was finally suppressed." The cult of Diana was still practiced in parts of sixteenth-century Italy where her followers assembled and "feasted and danced in her honor in order to insure the fertility of their fields" [7, 8].

A common method used by the Catholic Church to increase the conversion of "pagans" to Christianity was to discredit the traditional religions. This is illustrated as early as the tenth century by the canon Episcopi, an official church document. It described "certain wicked women who, deceived by Satan, believe themselves to join the train of the pagan goddess Diana during the night, and to cover great distances with a multitude of women riding on beasts, and during certain nights to be called to the service of their mistress." The canon then instructs that:

> The bishops and their ministers should by all means make great effort so that they may thoroughly eradicate the pernicious art of divination and magic, invented by the devil, from their parishes, and if they find any man or woman adhering to such a crime, they should reject them, turpidly dishonoured, from their parishes.

This was the beginning of the linking of traditional European religions to sorcery and witchcraft, a linkage that would become prominent over the following four centuries [9].

Another method used by the Catholic Church to discredit traditional religions was to link them to sexual excesses and sinful behavior. This was especially true of the cat-associated Norse goddess, Freya, who was also linked to both fertility and sexual behavior. The contrast between Freya and the Virgin Mary was stark, as noted by a historical account of Freya:

> Freyja's erotic qualities became an easy target for the new religion, in which an asexual virgin was the ideal woman … Freyja is called "a whore" and "a harlot" by the holy men and missionaries, whereas many of her functions in the everyday lives of men and women, such as protecting the vegetation and supplying assistance in childbirth, were transferred to the Virgin Mary [10].

Insofar as traditional goddesses like Diana, Isis, and Freya were becoming linked to Satan, it was merely a question of time before their associated cats would also be so linked. In *Witchcraft in the Middle Ages*, Jeffrey Russell cited an 1182 account as "one of the first times the Devil appears to his worshippers in the form of a cat." Saint Dominic (1170–1221), the founder of the Dominican Order, also taught that the Devil sometimes appeared as a black cat [11, 12].

It was Pope Gregory IX, however, who officially and definitively linked cats to the Devil. Trained as a lawyer, Gregory was a friend of Saint Dominic and was most concerned to confront the church's heresies when he became Pope in 1227. To gather information on heresies associated with the worship of Freya in Germany, Gregory appointed a local priest, Conrad of Marbury. Through the use of torture, Conrad elicited wild tales of Devil-worshippers holding orgies presided over by a large cat. Anxious to put down such heresies, Pope Gregory accepted the stories as truth and in 1233 issued an official papal bull, "Vox in Rama." In it he repeated some of Conrad's stories:

> Now this pestilence arises from the following beginnings. At first, a certain postulant [potential initiate] enters this school of perdition and is received. A kind of frog appears, which some are accustomed to call a toad. Some kiss it on its rear end and others give the damnable kiss on the mouth, receiving the tongue and saliva of the beast in their mouth. Along with the frog, sometimes a number of other animals are present, such as geese or ducks. These are often placed in an oven to bake. Then a thin pallid man comes forward to see the postulant. He appears like the skin drawn over bones that is left after some meat is consumed, and has the blackest of eyes. The postulant kisses him and feels cold and frigid. After the kiss, the memory of the Catholic faith completely disappears from his heart. They recline on couches during the banquet and they stand up when the meal is over. At this time, a black cat (gattus niger), the size of a small dog, with an upright tail descends backwards down a statue which is usually at the meeting. The postulant first kisses the cat's rear, then the master of the sect, and then other individuals in order who are worthy of the honor and perfect. Those who are imperfect and those not regarded as worthy, receive a word of peace from the master. Then, each member takes his place and after singing some songs, they face the cat in turn. The master says, "Save us" to the cat, and the one next to him states this. Then those present respond three times and say, "We know the master," and four times they say, "and we ought to obey you."
>   Following a sexual orgy a man then appears "from an obscure corner of the meeting." His upper body "shines with rays brighter than the sun" but his lower body "is hairy like a cat." This was Satan [13].

"Vox in Rama" urged the bishops to root out such heresies. "No vengeance against them is too harsh," according to Pope Gregory. "It is quite fitting that this pestilence be ground down as if by the pounding of the sea." Gregory then reminded the bishops that such actions were justified by the Bible, such as "zealous Elijah who put 450 prophets of Baal to the sword in the torrent of Kishon." Here, then, was an official death warrant for heretics and their cats. It would take cats 500 years to recover [13].

3.2   Cats During the Renaissance

At the same time as cats were valued for pest control during the Renaissance, they were otherwise held in low esteem and widely suspected of being associated with Satan. Indeed, the church had said that Satan often transformed himself into a cat and had therefore sanctioned their killing. Thus throughout Western Europe during the Renaissance, cats were tortured "to drive out the Devil," especially during Lent:

They were killed and buried in Oldenburg, Westphalia, Belgium, Switzerland and Bohemia; burnt on Shrove Tuesday in the Vosges, and in Alsace at Easter. In the Ardennes they were thrown into bonfires or roasted on the ends of long poles, or in wicker baskets on the first Sunday in Lent.

At Ypres during Lent, cats were thrown to their death from a high tower, a practice that continued until 1618. At Metz beginning in 1344, 13 cats were placed in an iron cage and burned, a practice that continued annually until 1777 [14–16].

The association of cats with Satan is also reflected in some paintings from the Renaissance period. A well-known example is Lorenzo Lotto's 1535 painting of "The Annunciation." Archangel Gabriel, with God the Father in the background, tells the Virgin Mary that she will give birth to a son. A cat, thought by many to represent Satan, flees in terror (Fig. 3.1). Art historian Caroline Bugler called this "one of the most memorable images of a feline ever produced." Another example is Domenico Ghirlandaio's 1481 painting of "The Last Supper." Judas is seated apart from the other Disciples across the table from Christ and a cat sits prominently at Judas' feet (Fig. 3.2). Renaissance artists portraying Adam and Eve in the Garden of Eden also "often added a cat to emphasize her insubordination" [17, 18].

Fig. 3.1 Lorenzo Lotto, "The Annunciation", 1534. Oil on canvas. As Archangel Gabriel tells the Virgin Mary that she will give birth to a son, a cat, thought to represent Satan, flees in terror. (Image courtesy of the Recanti Musei, Recanti, Italy)

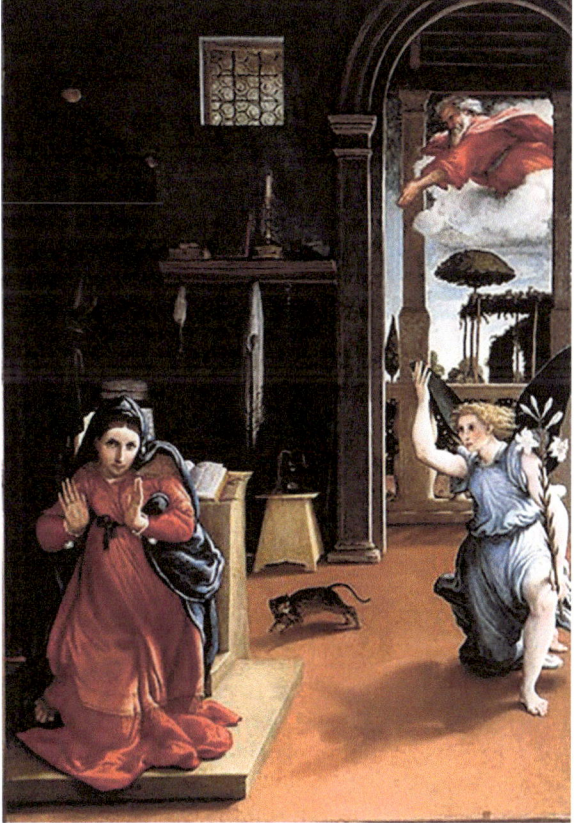

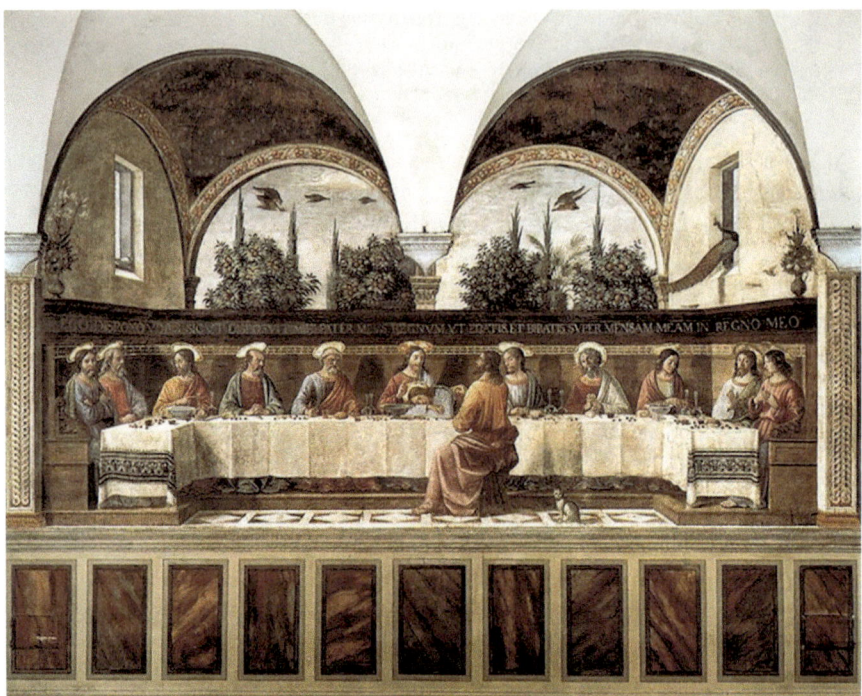

Fig. 3.2 Domenico Ghirlandiao, "The Last Supper", 1481, Fresco. Judas, seated apart from the other Disciples, has a cat, thought to represent Satan, sitting at his feet. (Image courtesy of Angelo Tartuferi, Director of Museo di San Marco, Florence, Italy)

The association of cats with Satan was strengthened following the bubonic plague of 1348–1349 which killed up to half the people in Europe. The population of England was reduced from 5 to 2.5 million. Some people believed that cats had caused the plague. For example, one document from the Inquisition described "a powder made from the body of a cat stuffed with herbs, grain and fruit, which is then hurled down from mountaintops in order to cause plague." In fact, the killing of cats probably made the plague more severe by allowing the rat population to increase [19].

The situation for cats grew even worse after 1400 when "witch hysteria" overtook Western Europe. Initially many animals were associated with witches, including cats, dogs, goats, wolves, rabbits, and toads, and "it was only in the later centuries when…cats were perceived as attractively exotic and mysterious, that they became the featured animal." In one of the first witch trials in Italy in 1424, a woman was said to have assumed the shape of a cat and had tried to kill her neighbor's child; she was burned at the stake. In the first witchcraft trial in England in 1566, a woman was said to have "a whytte spotted catte…[and they] feed the sayde catte with breade and milkye…and call it by the name of Satan." Accused of using sorcery to kill her husband, she was convicted and hanged [20–22].

Thus during the Renaissance period for the vast majority of the population, cats were thoroughly discredited. They continued to be used for pest control but were otherwise held in low esteem by most people. In his 1607 book *The History of the Four-Footed Beasts*, Edward Topsell described cats as "an unclean and impure beast that liveth only upon vermin and ravening." And William Shakespeare spoke for many when he wrote in *A Midsummer Night's Dream*: "Hang off, thou cat, thou burr! Vile thing, let loose, or I will shake thee from me like a serpent!" [23, 24].

3.3   The Beginning of Cat Rehabilitation

Remarkably, in the middle of the Renaissance period, at the time when the status of cats had reached its nadir, the rehabilitation of cats began. Major credit for this goes to Leonardo Da Vinci. According to art historian Stefano Zuffi, "Leonardo was fascinated by every aspect of nature, but he had a particular fondness for horses and cats." During the 1470s, when Leonardo was still in his 20s, he made a series of drawings of the Madonna with baby Jesus holding a cat. One of these appears to have been a sketch for an altarpiece, but it is not known whether it was ever painted. When Leonardo was in his 60s, he was still drawing cats, including a famous sketch of cats in different poses that hangs in Windsor Castle [25].

What is most unusual about Leonardo's interest in cats is that it occurred during the period when cats were being strongly associated with Satan and witches. In 1486 the *Malleus Maleficarum*, usually translated as the "Hammer of Witches," was published in Germany. This was the infamous book on witchcraft that was used by officials for identifying witches by means of torture; it recommended burning at the stake as the proper punishment. Yet even as this book was widely circulating, Leonardo was portraying a cat as a pet for Jesus. Increasingly over the next century, other European artists included cats in benign poses in their paintings, such as Germain Le Mannier's 1553 childhood portrait of the French King Charles IX holding a cat, Annibale Carracci's 1590 painting of two children playing with a cat, and Federico Barocci's 1580 painting the "Holy Family with a Cat" in which John the Baptist, as a child, plays with a cat as Mary, Joseph, and baby Jesus look on. By contrast, during this same period, many other artists were associating cats with evil.

Leonardo's drawings of baby Jesus holding a cat and subsequent paintings of children holding or playing with cats by other artists suggested that cats were occasionally being used as pets. Pet keeping at that time was a comparatively novel idea in Europe. In England it was strongly associated with royalty and the aristocratic ladies of the court. For example, King Richard II, who ruled from 1377 to 1399, kept a pet greyhound dog, even allowing it to sleep on his bed. Most of the earliest pet keeping, however, involved aristocratic ladies and small dogs. The noble women would carry them around and feed them from the table during meals. John Caius, a physician and naturalist, was the court physician to King Edward VI, Queen Mary, and Queen Elizabeth so had abundant opportunity to observe this practice. In his 1576 book *Of English Dogges*, Caius ridiculed the practice:

These dogges are little, pretty proper and fine, and sought for to satisfie the delicatenesse of folly for them to play and dally withal, to trifle away the treasures of time, to withdraw their minds from more commendable exercizes, and to content their corrupted concupiscences with vaine disport.

Such women, added Caius, "delight more in dogges that are deprived of all possibility of reason, than they do in children that be capable of wisdom and judgement" [26].

As an artist and scholar, Leonardo became one of the first of this group to support pet keeping. In a dissertation on "Late Medieval Pet Keeping," Kathleen Walker-Meikle described the importance of pets for writers at that time:

There is a great deal of evidence to suggest that pets, as portrayed in iconography, verse and letters, formed part of scholarly domestic life and these sources signify that the practice, which received little criticism, was widespread. The iconography suggests that pets became an artistic motif common to scholars, while verses written by scholars eulogizing their pets often received acclaim, and were widely imitated. The strong emotional attachment of scholars to their pets was not seen as an eccentricity but rather as a typical response to owning a companion animal.

Walker-Meikle cited not only published works and letters but also evidence from tombstones and especially "elegies and epitaphs written on the death of a pet, marking the owner's emotional attachment to the animals." In short, she concluded, "pet keeping was widespread among scholars" [27].

Although most of the writers cited by Walker-Meikle kept small dogs as pets, a few kept cats. For example, Italian poet Francesco Coppetta (1509–1553) wrote a lengthy elegy on the death of his cat, describing how "the cat would playfully bite his foot, leap on his chest and then go to sleep on his shoulder, presumably while the poet was writing at a desk." Joachim du Bellay (1522–1560), a prominent French Renaissance poet, wrote a poem lamenting the loss of his cat that had been allowed to sleep on his bed "and even steal from his master's plate." Italian poet Cesare Orsini (1571–1640) also wrote an epitaph to his dead cat, recalling how it "leaps into his lap with gentle paws, climbs up his shoulder, licks his face, purrs to the delight of his owner's ears, and playfully bites his hand." Thus according to Walker-Meikle, "owning a pet for a scholar is seen as a common occurrence, nothing to be commentated on, apart from possibly being eulogized in verse" [28].

An example of feline iconography from this period is Antonello da Messina's 1475 painting of "St. Jerome in His Study." St. Jerome, a fourth century theologian and historian, was credited with having translated the Bible into Latin. In the painting, St. Jerome is depicted reading at his desk with a cat lying quietly near his feet. According to Stefano Zuffi, placing the cat "alongside the scholarly saint is to fortify the alliance between intellectuals and cats." Walker-Meikle made the same point: "The presence of a pet in depictions of scholars portrays the social reality of widespread pet keeping by scholars, in keeping with their interior lifestyles…there is reason to think that it was a general phenomenon: that a pet was a normal accessory of a scholar in his study along with a desk, writing implements and books" [29, 30].

Another group that pioneered pet keeping in the late medieval period was the clergy. As Walker-Meikle noted, "It is fairly clear that pet keeping was a common feature of monastic life that was only occasionally officially condemned, and generally tolerated." This was said to be true "especially in nunneries." Dogs and small birds were the most common clerical pets, but cats were not rare and had the advantage of being justified to control rodents. Thus in about 1500, a long elegy was written on the death of a pet sparrow, killed by a cat at a Benedictine nunnery in England. Similarly, in a Dutch publication, a nun is shown spinning wool, while "a white cat catches and plays with the spool" [31].

According to Walker-Meikle, "the best evidence of the prevalence of pet keeping in religious orders is the constant criticism of the practice." An early fifteenth-century directive, for example, ordered that "cats, dogs, and other animals are not to be kept by nuns as they distract from seriousness." Indeed, the church was obligated to issue such directives even though it was aware that such prohibitions were being widely ignored. Officially the church was claiming that cats were associated with witches and Satan and was beginning to prosecute suspected witches. At the same time, many nuns were keeping cats as pets. James Serpell, in his book *In the Company of Animals*, suggested that "the only reason why the aristocracy and clergy were allowed to indulge in the same practice [of keeping cats as pets] was because they were quite literally above suspicion; their special status elevated them beyond the reach of public censure" [32–34].

The most important Renaissance clerical figure in England who was publicly associated with cats was Cardinal Thomas Wolsey (1473–1530), lord chancellor to King Henry VIII and the most important cleric in England after the archbishop of Canterbury. He was also regarded as the most powerful political figure after the king. Wolsey was described as "a great cat-lover [who] took his cats with him to important meetings, state dinners and church services." Similarly, William Laud (1573–1645), who was the archbishop of Canterbury and a senior advisor to King Charles I, was also a lover of cats and said to have been "one of the first people in England to import a tabby in the 1630s" [35, 36].

In summary, the Renaissance period in general was not a good time to have been a cat in Europe. Despite being used for pest control, cats were frequently abused and often killed. As the period progressed, a few cats became valued as pets by a small group of aristocrats, scholars, writers, and clergy. It was a modest beginning to what would become a markedly different relationship between cats and people. But it was a beginning.

3.4   Madness in the Renaissance

As had been true in the Middle Ages, occasional cases of madness continued to be described during the Renaissance. According to one scholar, people were considered to be mad if their behavior was "wild, extreme, violent or dangerous…Attacks on kith and kin were especially likely to be interpreted as evidence of insanity, as was self-violence and the destruction of personal property." Mentally disabled individuals were divided into "natural fools," also called idiots, who had been disabled from birth, and "non compes mentis," also called lunatics, who had developed mental illness later in life. Legal jurisdiction over idiots and lunatics in England was vested in the Court of Chancery until 1540 when it was transferred to the Court of Wards and Liveries [37].

Case histories of madness during this period were relatively few in number. Probably the best-known example was the case of Margery Kempe who came from an affluent family near Norfolk. Following the birth of her first child—she subsequently gave birth to 12 other children—she developed what today would be called postpartum psychosis with prominent auditory and visual hallucinations. She interpreted these as coming from God and in 1438, since she was not literate, sought out a priest who wrote down her story as *The Book of Margery Kempe*. This manuscript was rediscovered in 1934 and subsequently has been widely cited as the first English-language autobiography of a person with psychosis [38].

Another example of madness from this period was the psychosis of King Henry VI who ruled England from 1422 to 1453. He was described by historians as having been a weak and timid but well-meaning ruler. At the age of 31, he had a sudden onset of madness with "no known prodromal signs." The madness lasted for a year and a half during which time he also had neurological symptoms; for example "he could not walk or keep his head up." The king's maternal grandfather, King Charles VI of France, had also had intermittent episodes of madness during much of his reign [39].

An example of madness accompanied by violence was Peter Berchet, a law student in London. Over a period of several weeks in 1573, he exhibited increasingly strange behavior: "He rarely slept and would pace up and down in his room, striking himself upon his breast…and speaking softly to himself." Ultimately he stabbed a member of parliament thinking the man was someone else. Confined in the Tower of London, Berchet killed a guard and was then executed [40].

The most commonly assumed causes of madness during the Renaissance were physical. Thus Bartholomew de Sackville was said to be mad because of "a blow received on the head," and John Fitzwilliam's madness was dated to the time he had been "gravely ill." Consistent with such physical causes, most cases of madness were expected to eventually recover, as indicated by the fact that court-appointed guardians were only temporary [37].

As noted above, the Black Death and recurrent plagues that followed it decimated the population of England and Wales. By 1485 the total population had been reduced to 2.2. million but then it started to recover. By 1600 the total population had doubled but was disproportionately concentrated in urban areas. London, which had only 50,000 residents in 1500, had quadrupled in size to 200,000 by 1600. This meant that there were an increased number of mad people, including violent ones like Peter Berchet. Hospitals for mad people had become relatively common in Moslem countries, the first having been opened in Baghdad in the ninth century and the first in Europe opened in Moslem Spain in 1410.

The first, and for many years only, mental hospital in England was Bethlem. It was founded in 1247 in the Bishopsgate section of London as a religious priory and, like all such institutions, sheltered some individuals who were poor or sick. By the early 1400s, it had begun specializing in caring for mentally ill individuals and by 1598 had a census of 21 patients.

The year 1536 marked a major turning point for mad people in England. That year King Henry VIII, in an attempt to weaken the influence of the Catholic Church, began what became known as the dissolution of the monasteries. In addition to the regular churches, there were almost 900 other religious institutions—monasteries, convents, priories, and friaries—housing an estimated 12,000 people. Included in this group were many poor, elderly, and sick people, including mentally ill individuals who could not be managed at home. Some of these institutions were allowed to continue, such as the priory that became Bethlem Hospital, whose ownership was transferred from the church to the city of London. The majority of the institutions, however, were closed, leaving large numbers of poor and sick people with nowhere to go.

Even before the dissolution of the monasteries, mad people who had been released from Bethlem had been observed begging on the streets of London and surrounding villages. For most people begging was illegal in Tudor England, but those who had been in Bethlem were given a special badge allowing them to do so. Many of them adopted a distinctive dress, decorating themselves with multicolored ribbons, a foxtail, and a staff with streamers. These people were widely known as Tom O'Bedlam and Bess O'Bedlam. Since they had a legal right to beg, other people also created false badges, adopted their dress, and begged on the streets.

In the second half of the nineteenth century, following the dissolution of the monasteries, mentally ill beggars became a much more common sight in England. One measure of this was the number of ballads written about them. Such ballads were printed on single sheets or "broadsides" and sold for a penny apiece. The ballads could be read (approximately half of London's males were literate at that time), or they could be sung in the streets or at fairs and were "the cheapest and probably the most widely distributed form of popular literature of the time" [41, 42].

According to a historian of English popular culture, "amongst many individual songs and verses, two principal song-families stand out: 'Bedlamite verses' and 'mad songs'." Many of them featured Tom O'Bedlam:

From forth my sad and darksome cell,
And from the deep abyss of hell
Poor Tom is come to view the world again,
To see if he can ease distempered brain.
Fear and despair possess his soul,
Hark how the angry furies howl!

Bishop Thomas Percy claimed in 1763 that "the English had more songs and ballads on the subject of insanity than of their neighbors…We certainly do not find the same in the printed collections of French and Italian songs." And according to David Mellett, "It would be a logical assumption to consider them [Bedlamite songs] as evidence of contemporary popular imagery, and an imagery which they reinforced as well as reflected" [42, 43].

In summary, until the end of the Renaissance period in England, most people in England, except for a small group of artists, writers, and clergy, continued to link cats to Satan. There was also no indication that the incidence of madness exceeded the baseline rate, as described in Chap. 1, of 0.5 per 1000 population associated with cerebral infections, brain trauma, nutritional deficiencies, etc. Bethlem Hospital, England's only mental hospital, housed only 21 patients. But all this was about to change.

References

1. Engels D. Classical cats: the rise and fall of the sacred cat. New York: Routledge; 1999. p. 93.
2. Simpson F. The book of the cat. London: Cassell; 1903. p. 6.
3. Tabor R. Cats: the rise of the cat. London: BCA; 1991. p. 36.
4. Summers WH. The rise and spread of Christianity in Europe. London: Butler and Tanner; 1897. p. 112–3.
5. Tabor R. Cats: the rise of the cat. London: BCA; 1991. p. 14. See also the entry on Freya on Wikipedia. https://en.wikipedia.org/wiki/Freyja.
6. Summers WH. The rise and spread of Christianity in Europe. London: Butler and Tanner; 1897. p. 82, 102, 103.
7. Engels D. Classical cats: the rise and fall of the sacred cat. New York: Routledge; 1999. p. 140–2.
8. Russell JB. Witchcraft in the middle ages. Ithaca: Cornell University Press; 1972. p. 48.
9. Russell JB. Witchcraft in the middle ages. Ithaca: Cornell University Press; 1972. p. 80. See also the Wikipedia entry on canon Episcopi.
10. Nasstrom B-M. Freyha, The great goddess of the North, quoted in the Wikipedia entry on Freya.
11. Russell JB. Witchcraft in the middle ages. Ithaca: Cornell University Press; 1972. p. 131.
12. Engels D. Classical cats: the rise and fall of the sacred cat. New York: Routledge; 1999. p. 157.
13. Engels D. Classical cats: the rise and fall of the sacred cat. New York: Routledge; 1999. p. 183–5.
14. Zeuner, FE. A history of domesticated animals. London: Hutchinson; 1963. p. 397.
15. Winslow HM. Concerning cats. Boston: Lothrop; 1900. p. 207.
16. Kete K. The beast in the boudoir. Berkeley: University of California Press; 1994. p. 119.
17. Bugler C. The cat: 3,500 years of the cat in art. New York: Merrell; 2011. p. 275.
18. Tabor R. Cats: the rise of the cat. London: BCA; 1991. p. 137.
19. Russell JB. Witchcraft in the middle ages. Ithaca: Cornell University Press; 1972. p. 240.
20. Russell JB. Witchcraft in the middle ages. Ithaca: Cornell University Press; 1972. p. 216, 234.
21. Tabor R. Cats: the rise of the cat. London: BCA; 1991. p. 52.
22. Clutten-Brock J. Cats: ancient and madness. Cambridge: Harvard University Press; 1993. p. 55.
23. Thomas K. Man and the natural world. New York, Oxford; 1983. p. 109.
24. Shakespeare W. A midsummer night's dream, Act III, ii.
25. Zuffi S. The cat in art. New York: Abrams; 2007. p. 98.
26. Swabe J. Animals, disease, and human society. New York: Routledge; 1999. p. 162–3.
27. Walker-Meikle K. Late medieval pet keeping: gender, status and emotions. Ann Arbor: University Microfilms International; 2013. p. 119–20.
28. Walker-Meikle K. Late medieval pet keeping: gender, status and emotions. Ann Arbor: University Microfilms International; 2013. p. 146, 151, 145, 153.
29. Zuffi S. The cat in art. New York: Abrams; 2007. p. 85.
30. Walker-Meikle K. Late medieval pet keeping: gender, status and emotions. Ann Arbor: University Microfilms International; 2013. p. 162.

31. Walker-Meikle K. Late medieval pet keeping: gender, status and emotions. Ann Arbor: University Microfilms International; 2013. p. 108, 111, 110, 104.
32. Walker-Meikle K. Late medieval pet keeping: gender, status and emotions. Ann Arbor: University Microfilms International; 2013. p. 103, 107.
33. Tabor R. Cats: the rise of the cat. London: BCA; 1991. p. 56.
34. Serpell J. In the company of animals. Oxford: Basil Blackwell; 1986. p. 46.
35. Bugler C. The cat: 3,500 years of the cat in art. New York: Merrell; 2011. p. 200.
36. MacDonogh K. Reigning cats and dogs: a history of pets at court since the renaissance. New York: Saint Martin's Press; 1999. p. 207.
37. Neugebauer R. Medieval and early modern theories of mental illness. Arch Gen Psychiatry. 1979;36(4):477–83. https://doi.org/10.1001/archpsyc.1979.01780040119013.
38. Craun M. The story of Margery Kempe. Psychiatr Serv. 2005;56:655–6.
39. Clarke B. Mental disorder in early Britain. Cardiff: University of Wales Press; 1975. p. 177–8.
40. Chermely C. Some faces of madness in Tudor England. Historian. 1987;49:309–28.
41. Mellett DJ. The prerogative of asylumdom. New York: Garland; 1982.
42. Wiltonburg J. Madness and society in the street ballads of early modern England. Journal of Popular Culture. 1988;21:101–27.
43. Mellett DJ. The prerogative of asylumdom. New York: Garland; 1982. p. 87.

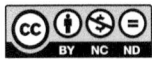

The Rise of Cats and Madness: II. The Seventeenth and Eighteenth Centuries

4

4.1 The Continuing Persecution of Cats

Seventeenth-century England witnessed an increasing interest in pet keeping, initially confined to the aristocracy but later extending to the expanding middle class. The keeping of cats as pets was still unusual except for a small group of intellectuals, artists, writers, and clerics. By the eighteenth century, prominent intellectuals such as Samuel Johnson and Horace Walpole were well known as cat lovers, adding respectability to this choice of pet. The seventeenth century also saw a sharp rise in public interest in madness. It became a major theme of the Elizabethan and Jacobean stage. Bethlem Hospital became an increasing magnet for visitors, and the number of psychiatric beds, both public and private, began to rapidly increase. By the mid-eighteenth century, Bethlem was widely regarded as a human zoo, attracting up to 19,000 visitors annually to observe its 200 mad inmates. For many writers, such as Jonathan Swift, madness became a dominant theme, and an unusual number of poets, who had pioneered the keeping of cats as pets, were themselves experiencing madness. By the end of the century, madness had become known as "the English malady," and it was being widely debated whether madness was increasing.

The seventeenth century was not kind to the people of England. During one 24-year period, from 1642 to 1666, the English Civil Wars were fought with upward of 200,000 casualties from fighting and disease; King Charles I was convicted of treason and beheaded; another visitation of plague killed an estimated 100,000 people in London, almost a quarter of the population; and the Great Fire of London destroyed 70,000 of the 80,000 homes in the central city.

The seventeenth century was also not kind to the cats of England or to their owners, some of whom were thought to be witches. Between 1565, when the first major witchcraft trial took place in England, and 1716, when Mary Hicks and her 9-year-old daughter were convicted of witchcraft, it has been estimated that approximately 500 witches were condemned to death. In many cases the evidence against the accused, two thirds of whom were elderly women, included that she had a special relationship with an animal called a "familiar". Cats were most commonly cited

© E. Fuller Torrey 2022
E. F. Torrey, *Parasites, Pussycats and Psychosis*,
https://doi.org/10.1007/978-3-030-86811-6_4

although dogs, birds, toads, and other animals could also be "familiars". In his book on witchcraft trials in Europe, Geoffrey Scarre claimed that accusations of the use of cats and other familiars were more common in England than in other parts of Europe [1].

From a feline point of view, the century started very badly. Following the 1603 death of Queen Elizabeth, the last of the Tudors, James I was appointed king of England. As the king of Scotland, James had been convinced that witches had tried to kill him, and in 1597 he had published a book on *Daemonology*, emphasizing the dangers of witchcraft. Included in the book was an account of a 1590 trial in which an accused witch had confessed to having sacrificed a cat in her effort to kill the king. Thus, when James I took the throne in England, he changed a 1563 law and made witchcraft punishable by death [2].

A century of witch-hunting ensued. One of the first major trials took place in 1612 at Pendle Hill in Lancaster where ten women and two men were accused of murdering ten people by witchcraft. One of the accused died in prison, one was found not guilty, and the other ten were executed by hanging. Such trials peaked in 1644–1646 in East Anglia where Matthew Hopkins appointed himself as "witch finder general" and went from town to town, identifying the local witches for a fee. He is thought to have been responsible for the deaths of as many as 300 women [3].

During these same years, cats continued to be persecuted because of their connection to Satan. For example, on New Year's Day in 1638 in the Ely Cathedral, "there was a great noise and disturbance near the choir occasioned by the roasting of a live cat tied to a spit…in the presence of a large and boisterous crowd". Later in the century, when anti-Catholic sentiment had become widespread, "it was the practice to stuff the burning effigies [of the Pope] with live cats so that their screams might add dramatic effect". At many county fairs, "a popular sport was that of shooting a cat suspended in a basket" [4].

4.2   Pet Keeping Becomes More Popular

At the same time as cats and witches were being persecuted in the seventeenth century, pet keeping in general was becoming more widespread. As stated by Keith Thomas in *Man and the Natural World*, "It was in the sixteenth and seventeenth centuries that pets seemed to have really established themselves as a normal feature of the middle-class household, especially in the towns, where animals were less likely to be functional necessitates…Pets were company for the lonely, relaxation for the tired, a compensation for the childless" [5].

The array of animals that were kept as pets was remarkably varied. Dogs were by far the most common, but in addition there were pet monkeys, tortoises, otters, rabbits, squirrels, and, on farms, pet lambs. Pet birds were especially popular and widely available in London bird markets. These included canaries, nightingales, goldfinches, larks, linnets, parrots, magpies, jackdaws, jays, thrushes, starlings, bullfinches, wrens, and cuckoos. The common characteristics of all pets that distinguished them from non-pet animals were that they were given a name, they were allowed in the house, and they were often taken to church. According to Thomas, "there was an official dog-whipper in almost every church and one of the main purposes of the Laudian communion rails was to keep dogs away from the alter" [6].

As pet keeping was spreading to the middle class in the seventeenth century, encouragement of the practice continued to come from the top. James I, who ruled from 1603 to 1625, had two favorite hounds, one of which was unfortunately shot by his wife when she mistook it for a deer. The king was accused "of loving his dogs more than his subjects". Charles I (1625 to 1649) also kept many dogs, and "his wife gave birth prematurely in 1628 after being involved in a fight between large dogs". Charles II (1660–1685) had spaniels which now bear his name; they were said to overrun the palace "causing one courtier to remark, 'God save your Majesty, but God damn your dogs.'" The grand homes of the English aristocracy were similarly often overrun by dogs and other pets. In one home in 1638, it was said that "the great hall was strewn with marrow bones and swarmed with hawks, hounds, spaniels and terriers…In the parlor favored dogs lay around the hearth…By the late seventeenth century polite society was coming to despise this old way of housekeeping 'with dogs' turds and marrow-bones as ornaments in the hall." [7, 8]

In addition to royalty and the aristocracy, the English upper class also set the social standard for pet keeping. An example was Samuel Pepys, the son of a tailor, graduate of Cambridge, member of parliament, and chief secretary to the Admiralty under Charles II and James II. Pepys kept a pet monkey and a canary and admitted to being "much troubled" when the latter died. Pepys wife also had a dog, and in a 1660 entry in his famous diary, he noted one of the timeless problems of pet keeping: "So to bed, where my wife and I had some high words upon my telling her that I would fling the dog which her brother gave her out of the window if he pissed in the house anymore" [8, 9].

4.3   Cats as Pets

Despite the increasingly widespread practice of pet keeping in seventeenth century England, keeping a cat as a pet continued to be unusual. It wasn't that cats were not present; indeed, they were numerous, especially in London and smaller cities where they helped to control the mouse and rat population. This is verified by accounts of the Great Plague which describes dogs and cats dead in the streets from the disease. Also, during England's civil wars, there is an account of royalist forces being besieged in Colchester "until they were reduced to killing cats for food" [10].

The few examples of cat pet keeping at this time mostly involved aristocrats, clerics, poets, and artists. For example, Frances Teresa Stuart, a distant relative of the royal family, was said by Samuel Pepys to be the most beautiful woman he had ever seen; she had refused King Charles II's offer to become his mistress and instead married the duke of Richmond. She kept cats as pets and, just prior to her death in 1702, "bequeathed a legacy for the upkeep of her cats". Robert Herrick, a seventeenth century English poet and cleric, kept a cat as a pet along with a dog, sparrow, pet lamb, and pig, the last of which "was taught to drink beer out of a tankard".

Similarly, in France, Antoinette Deshoulieres, a well-known seventeenth century poet at the court of Louis XIV, "wrote epistles to her friends and their cats under the name of her cat, Grisette". And Mademoiselle Dupuy, an acclaimed harpist, credited her cats with her musical success and at her death left her estate, including two houses, to her cats "with meticulous directions on how their meals were to be served". The court voided the will and awarded the estate to her relatives [11, 12].

But it was the artists in England who initially provided visual permission to keep a cat as a pet. The way had been paved by the Dutch school of genre painting in which cats were depicted as part of the household in scenes from everyday life. Several Dutch artists also depicted children playing with cats, including Jan Steen who painted at least four such scenes. Such scenes were still very unusual in European art. In his book *Cats: The Rise of the Cat*, Roger Tabor contended that, based on paintings at this time, the dog was "at least ten times more popular than the cat" [13].

Possibly inspired by the Dutch school, between 1665 and 1670, Mary Beale painted a portrait of a young girl holding a cat (Fig. 4.1). Beale was the daughter of a clergyman and was regarded as England's first successful female portrait painter. She was prominent in London intellectual circles and was personal friends with

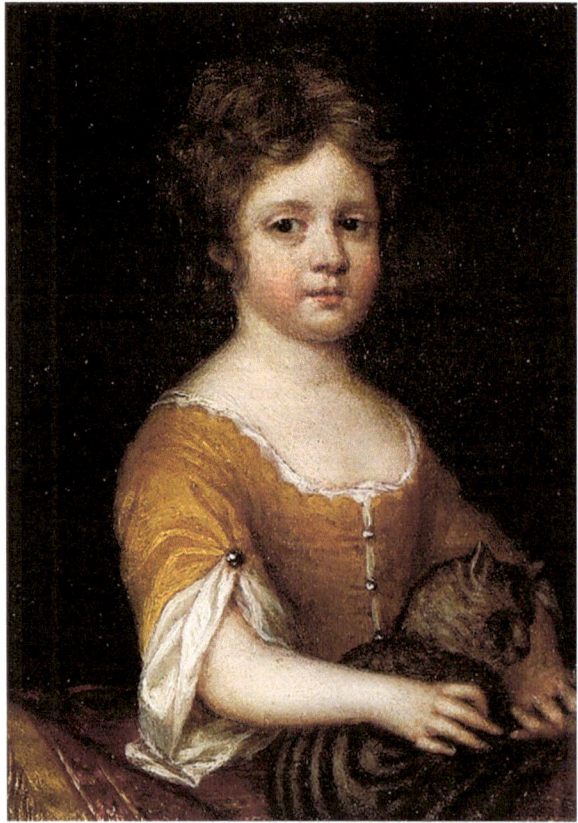

Fig. 4.1 Mary Beale, "Portrait of a Girl with a Cat", c. 1665-1670, Oil on vellum. The inclusion of a cat in a portrait is very unusual in British art at this time. (Image courtesy of West Suffolk Heritage Service, under the Creative Commons License Attribution (CC BY-NC-ND))

many clerics, including the archbishop of Canterbury. As art historian Caroline Bugler noted, the inclusion of a cat in a portrait is "unusual in British art of this period". What makes it even more unusual was that Mary Beale had grown up in Suffolk in East Anglia and would have been a teenager during the East Anglia witch trials of 1644–1646. She certainly would have been aware of the common beliefs about cats. The fact that she chose to ignore them and depict a cat as an appropriate pet for a young child was certainly unusual but a harbinger of things to come [14].

4.4   Increasing Interest in Madness

The early years of the seventeenth century in England witnessed a striking increase in the public's interest in madness. The earliest manifestations had been seen in the closing years of the sixteenth century as beggars from Bethlem Hospital appeared on the streets, as discussed in the previous chapter. According to Michael MacDonald in *Mystical Bedlam*, "During the late sixteenth and early seventeenth centuries, the English people became more concerned about the prevalence of madness, gloom and self-murder than they had ever been before and the reading public developed a strong fascination with classical medical psychology…Interest in insanity quickened about 1580, and madmen, melancholics, and suicides became familiar literary types. Scientific writers popularized medical lore about melancholy and clergymen wrote treatises about consoling the troubled in mind" [15].

The increasing interest in madness in sixteenth-century England was perhaps most clearly in evidence on the Elizabethan and Jacobean stage. Newly opened London theatres, such as the Curtain, Rose, and Globe, attracted a thousand or more patrons each afternoon who, for a penny admission, were entertained by the latest productions. As Thomas Dalby noted in a detailed analysis of this period, "the depiction of madness was ubiquitous during plays of this time". Similarly in *The History of Bethlem*, Jonathan Andrews et al. observed: "For some reason, the first quarter of the seventeenth century was a period in which playwrights seem first to have 'discovered' Bethlem as a dramatic resource". And in *Mystical Bedlam*, Michael MacDonald claimed that "the Jacobean stage teemed with idiots and lunatics" [16–18].

William Shakespeare (1564–1616) is of course the best known of these playwrights. According to Dalby, "in at least 20 of his 38 plays (and many of his sonnets) he comments on the nature of madness and its causes". The title character of *Hamlet*, written in 1601, has received extensive psychiatric analysis; Joseph Collins suggested that "the mentality of the latter [Hamlet] has probably occupied more printed space than that of any other person, real or imaginary". Opinions regarding whether Hamlet was feigning insanity or was truly insane have been approximately evenly divided, with many prominent psychiatric professionals having written on the subject. *King Lear* has also elicited considerable professional interest, both for the apparent dementia in the 80-year-old king and for the feigned madness of Edgar when he disguises himself as a mad Tom O'Beldam [19].

Other Elizabethan and Jacobean playwrights who used madness prominently include the following:

- *Robert Greene* (1558–1592): In *The History of Orlando Furioso*, a man becomes mad, kills a king, and later recovers his sanity after being treated by a witch.
- *Thomas Kyd* (1558–1594): In *The Spanish Tragedy*, which was very popular at the time, a man and his wife both become mad when they learn that their son is dead.
- *Christopher Marlowe* (1564–1593): In *Tamburlaine*, a woman becomes mad when she discovers that her husband has killed himself.
- *Thomas Dekker* (1572–1632): In *The Honest Whore*, one scene is set in Bethlem Hospital and introduces three madmen. In *Match Me in London*, a woman feigns madness.
- *Ben Johnson* (1572–1637): In *Bartholomew Fair*, a woman is told that she must marry a madman so she visits Bethlem to assess prospective husbands.
- *John Fletcher* (1579–1625): In *The Mad Lover*, a man becomes mad when he is rejected by a woman but regains his sanity when she later marries him. In *The Two Noble Kinsmen*, a woman becomes mad. In *The Pilgrim* some of the play is set in Bethlem.
- *John Webster* (1580–1634): In *The Duchess of Malfi*, a man attempts to drive his sister mad by having her watch madmen. Instead the man himself later becomes mad. *Northward Ho*, written with Thomas Dekker, includes a scene set in Bethlem.
- *Thomas Middleton* (1580–1627): In *The Changeling*, one scene is set in a private madhouse, and the doctor running it is also said to be mad.
- *Philip Massinger* (1583–1640): In *A Very Woman*, a man and his lover both become mad. In *A New Way to Pay Old Debts*, a man becomes mad and is treated by doctors from Bethlem.
- *John Ford* (1586–1640): In *Broken Heart*, a woman becomes mad, and in *The Lover's Melancholy*, a man becomes mad.

This outpouring of mad characters in the plays of the late Elizabethan and Jacobean period is remarkable and was without precedent at the time. What might explain it? In *The History of Bethlem*, Andrews et al. suggested a possible explanation for the prominence of Bethlem Hospital in these plays. Two of the theaters in which the plays were being featured were physically located close to Bethlem Hospital as well as to the Artillery Gardens, where fireworks were shown, and to the Tower of London. Thus visitors to Bethlem would be likely to also be interested in plays about madness, forming "a natural extension to the round of pleasure". Another explanation was suggested by Robert Reed in his book *Bedlam on the Jacobean Stage*. "The antics of mad folk, if embellished, were particularly suitable to the stage" claimed Reed. In short, madness made good theater [20, 21].

Perhaps the simplest explanation is that madness was a prominent theme in the plays at that time because it was of great interest to the public. The playwrights and theatres were very competitive and tended to cater to the interest of their audience. As noted above, the public's interest in madness significantly increased in the latter part of the sixteenth century. It seemed to some people that madness was increasing, an idea expressed in several plays. For example, in *The Honest Whore*, the sweeper at Bethlem Hospital claimed that "if all the mad folk…should come hither, there would not be left ten men in the city". Shakespeare also expressed this idea in Act V of Hamlet:

- Hamlet: How long has thou been a grave maker?
- First Clown: Of all the days in the year, I came to't that day that our last king Hamlet overcame Fortinbras.
- Hamlet: How long is that since?
- First Clown:…it was the very day that young Hamlet was born; he that is mad, and sent into England.
- Hamlet: Ay, marry, why was he sent into England?
- First Clown: Why, because he was mad; he shall recover his wits there; or, if he do not, 'tis no great matter there.
- Hamlet: Why?
- First Clown: Twill not be seen in him there; there the men are as mad as he.

Subsequent events would support this idea.

4.5   Bethlem as a Human Zoo

The plays of the late Elizabethan and Jacobean period suggest that by the early 1600s Bethlem had become well known in London. This is confirmed by a 1610 account of a visit by Lord Henry Percy, 9th earl of Northumberland, who "saw the lions, the shew of Bethlem…and the fireworks of the Artillery Gardens". The lions were being exhibited at the Tower of London, the city's first zoo. According to Michael DePorte's *Nightmares and Hobbyhorses*, at this time Bethlem "was commonly regarded less as a hospital than as a kind of zoo, with a fine, permanent exhibition of human curiosities". In addition to usually being able to observe mad people, visitors to Bethlem could listen to "cryings, screechings, roarings, brawlings, shakings of chains, swearings, frettings, [and] chaffings". As summarized by Edward O'Donoghue in his history of Bethlem Hospital, "Everybody who lived in London or ever came to London visited Bethlem as a matter of course" [22–25].

At the beginning of the seventeenth century, when regular visits to Bethlem began, the hospital only had 21 patients. By 1632 this number had increased to 27 patients and by 1642 to 44 as London's population increased. Mid-century visitors included the two most prominent diarists of their era; John Evelyn went out of curiosity to see something "extraordinary," and Samuel Pepys took his cousin's children who were visiting from Cambridge. By this time problems associated with visiting had apparently gotten out of control, so the hospitals' governors implemented restrictions on Sunday visiting, restricted the length of visits, and decreed that "noe Lunaticker that lyeth naked…[can] be seene by any [visitor]…without the Consent of the Physician". Such rules were largely ignored [26, 27].

By the 1670s Bethlem had become severely overcrowded. The hospital governors therefore agreed to build a new hospital to accommodate 120 patients since the present hospital was said to be "very old weak and ruinous and too small and straight for keeping the greater number of Lunatiker as are therein at present and more are often needful to be sent thither". The new hospital, opened in 1676, was a magnificent building modeled on French architectural principles and widely referred to as a palace for lunatics. Some people even speculated that the building was so attractive that it "might encourage exaltation and make everybody half mad—in order to be a lodger there" [28, 29].

The new building made the visitor-associated problems even worse since visitors now wished to come to see the building as well as the mad people. A year after the new hospital opened, a report of the hospital's governors noted "persistent complaints of prostitutes and thieves infiltrating the ranks of visitors" as well as visitors getting patients drunk "while hucksters hawked Nutts Cake [and] fruite to the patients and visitors, contributing to the fairground atmosphere". Four years later the governors noted "the greate quantity of persons that come daily to see the said Lunatikes". Representative was James Yonge, a visitor from Plymouth, who came to see "all that was curious in London" [30].

One way in which Bethlem's governors tried to prevent overcrowding was to restrict admissions to patients thought to be curable. Thus no patients with mental retardation or who had been mentally ill for a long period of time were admitted. Admissions were accepted for a period of up to 1 year, and, if the patients had not improved by that time, most were discharged as incurable. Thus there were very few long stay patients at Bethlem until new wings were added for such patients in the eighteenth century [31].

Among the better-known patients in Bethlem at this time were James Carkesse and Nathaniel Lee. Carkesse had graduated from Oxford, was a fellow of the Royal Society, and had worked under Samuel Pepys in the naval office. He then became delusional, believing himself to be the victim of a plot, and was hospitalized. He is remembered today for the poetry he wrote while confined and that was later published. He insisted that he was not mad but rather that his poetic genius was being mistaken for madness. Nathaniel Lee had been a leading English playwright and poet before becoming mentally ill. Famously, he described his hospitalization as follows: "They called me mad, and I called them mad, and damn them, they outvoted me" [32–34].

By the closing years of the seventeenth century, voices began to be raised against using Bethlem as a human freakshow. For example, in 1689, Thomas Tyron called for the closing of Bethlem to visitors. He argued that it was "a very Undecent, Inhumane thing" for the governors of the hospital "to make...a Show of those Unhappy Objects of Charity committed to their care (by exposing them, and naked too perhaps of either Sex) to the Idle Curiosity of every vain Boy, petulant Wench, or Drunken Companion". Tyron also claimed that many people regarded as sane in England were in fact behaving in ways that were just as "mad" as the inmates of Bethlem:

"Is it worse for men to sit playing with straws than to become drunkards who 'swallow down vast Estates at their Throats, and Piss away the Labours of their Ancestors against the Wall"? What then is the world, he asks, but "a great Bedlam, where those that are more mad lock up those that are less"?

It would be almost a century before Tyron's suggestion of closing Bethlem to visitors would be taken seriously [35].

4.6   Was Madness Increasing?

The fascination of seventeenth-century Londoners with madness was striking. First, there was an outpouring of plays featuring mad characters and Bethlem Hospital itself. That was followed by thousands of people each year visiting the hospital to observe mad people. The exhibiting of mad people was not unique to London; it was also done at the Bicetre Hospital in Paris and at the Pennsylvania Hospital in Philadelphia, the latter having been influenced by Bethlem. But at no other place in the world was there a fascination with madness at this time such as there was in England. As Michael MacDonald summarized it, "Madness was on men's lips in the seventeenth century" [36].

Another indication of the interest in mental illness in seventeenth-century England was the enthusiastic reception for Robert Burton's *The Anatomy of Melancholy*. Burton, a clergyman and scholar, first published the 900 page book in 1621 and then republished it four more times over the next 17 years. By "melancholy" Burton included not only depression but virtually all other forms of mental illness except violent madness. At this time melancholy was widely understood to be "the first stage of madness". Burton himself emphasized the diversity of symptoms of melancholy: "The tower of Babel never yielded such confusion of tongues as the chaos of melancholy doth variety of symptoms…The character of a melancholy man is more changeable than Proteus". Elsewhere Burton claimed that "madness is simply melancholy turned violent". Burton's book would remain popular for two centuries and was a favorite of Samuel Johnson [37, 38].

It was also at this time that the first comprehensive treatise on suicide was published. In 1630 William Gouge, a Puritan cleric, claimed that suicide was on the increase:

I suppose that scarce an age since the beginning of the world hath afforded more examples of this desperate inhumanity, than this our present age; and that of all sorts of people, clergy, laity, learned, unlearned, noble, mean, rich, poor, free, bond, male, female, young and old. It is therefore high time that the danger of this desperate, devilish and damnable practice be plainly and fully set out [39].

The seventeenth century also witnessed an increasing need for psychiatric hospital beds in England. Previously most people suffering from madness had been able to be kept at home or boarded out to a family that was paid for the service by local authorities. Such arrangements no longer seemed sufficient. In London in 1600, when the city's population was approximately 200,000, Bethlem Hospital had 21 beds. In 1676 the city's population was about 500,000 when the new hospital opened with 120 beds. Thus the supply of psychiatric beds was increasing much faster than the population.

Additional psychiatric beds were made available by the opening of private madhouses, especially in London. According to Michael MacDonald's *Mystical Bedlam*, "Beginning about 1660 scores of entrepreneurs founded private madhouses to care for the insane". Private madhouses were also being opened elsewhere in Europe at this time, especially in France, "yet nowhere did they appear in such profusion as in England or play such a dominant role". Such facilities varied in size and were completely unregulated until the end of the eighteenth century [40, 41].

Some of the private madhouses were owned and operated by physicians, others by clerics or other laypersons. For example, Thomas Allen, a physician at Bethlem, also ran a private madhouse at Finsbury. James Carkesse, who had been a patient at Bethlem, was later hospitalized at Dr. Allen's madhouse. John Ashbourne, an Anglican minister, ran a private madhouse in Suffolk, and "in 1661 he was slain by one of his charges". Conditions in these facilities were often marginal, as demonstrated by Dr. Allen giving James Carkesse a cat to control the mice and rats in his cell [42, 43].

The one thing that all the private madhouses offered was privacy. No records or reports were kept so cases of madness could be discretely hidden away by a family, in contrast to Bethlem where visitors could see them. One consequence of this privacy is that we have no data on how many mad people were so hospitalized or what their diagnoses were. We know, for example, that by 1724 there were 15 private madhouses in London alone, but we don't know how many patients were in each. Therefore, assessing the true prevalence of madness at this time is very difficult [44].

In summary, in seventeenth-century England, pet keeping became more common, with a few people even keeping cats as pets despite the ongoing persecution of witches. There was also a significant increased interest in madness and need for more psychiatric beds, especially in London. Was this an aberration or a trend? The eighteenth century would answer this question.

4.7   Cats in Eighteenth Century England

In *Man and the Natural World*, Keith Thomas observed that "in the eighteenth century the domestic cat established itself as a creature to be cosseted and cherished for its companionship". There were several reasons for this. One, according to Thomas, was that "the cat gained in popularity as standards of domestic cleanliness rose" since cats are perpetually cleaning themselves. Another reason was the arrival of the brown (also called gray) rat in Europe. Until the seventeenth century, Europe had been inhabited by only the black rat. However, the brown rat was stronger, multiplied more rapidly, and was more difficult to control. By the eighteenth century, the brown rat had established itself in England and was spreading across Northern Europe. The value of cats for rat control became much more important as "many administrative authorities began to set aside a special budget for the breeding and maintenance of ratting cats in museums, libraries, prisons, barracks, warehouses and stores" [45, 46].

Yet another reason for the elevated status of cats in the eighteenth century was the expansion of the English economy and growth of the middle class. As the economy improved, so did the number of merchants, shopkeepers, tradesmen, clerks, and skilled craftsmen, often with money to spare. There was said to be "an almost frenzied propensity to consume," especially novel products that were being introduced from England's overseas territories. The imports included new and improved varieties of sheep, cattle, horses, pigs, dogs, and even cats, such as the exotic long-haired Angora cat which was imported from Turkey. The rising middle class also aspired to be like the upper class which, as described previously, had set the standards for pet keeping [47].

Perhaps the most important reason for the enhanced status of cats in eighteenth-century England was the decline in belief in witchcraft, especially among the educated class. In 1711 Joseph Addison published an essay in the *Spectator* ridiculing witchcraft "as a medieval superstition". Implicitly this helped to sever the popular association between cats and witches. It is even possible that some educated people then began to keep cats as a badge of their sophisticated status. Among the uneducated, however, the belief in witches died more slowly. The last witches to be tried in England were Jane Wenham in 1712 in Hertfordshire and Mary Hicks and her 9-year-old daughter in 1716 in Huntingdon. Wenham was convicted by a jury, but the clearly skeptical judge set aside her conviction and released her. During her trial one of her accusers had claimed that Jane Wenham could fly, and the judge had observed that there was no law against flying. Mary Hicks and her daughter, however, did not fare as well; they were both convicted of witchcraft and hung. Finally, in 1735 the witch-finding era in England came to an official end with the passing by parliament of the Witchcraft Act; this made it a crime to accuse anyone of witchcraft with a penalty of up to 1-year imprisonment [48, 49].

The increasing popularity of cats as pets in the eighteenth century, however, was specific to certain groups of people. According to Kathleen Kete's *The Beast in the Boudoir*, "the cat was linked rather with bohemia"—artists, poets, writers, and other intellectuals. "The companionship of a like-minded animal became a trope of intellectuals, the cat a sign for the literary life". In England, as in France, "a pronounced taste for cats in certain people was an indication of superior merit". Francois-Rene Chateaubriand, a French historian and politician, stated it as follows: "What I like about the cat is his character, independent and almost heartless, which prevents him from attaching himself to anyone…The cat lives alone, he has no need of society" [50].

Although bohemians and intellectuals were embracing the cat at this time, the embrace did not extend to the lower class. Georges-Louis Buffon's popular book on natural history, translated into English in 1785, characterized cats as "cruel and rapacious animals…they are all destructive, ferocious and untamable". The persecution of cats also continued; this is illustrated by Williams Hogarth's 1751 engravings on "The Four Stages of Cruelty" in which several boys are depicted torturing cats, including throwing one out of a window. In France at this time, the Great Cat Massacre took place in which young apprentices in a print shop, tired of seeing their master treat his cat better than themselves, beat to death the master's cat and all the other cats in the neighborhood [51].

4.8   Cats in Art and Poetry

The evolving eighteenth-century attitude toward cats is also illustrated by their place in art and poetry. Art historian Caroline Bugler noted that "the eighteenth century witnessed a growing tenderness towards the cat in literature and art, as befitted an age of sensibility…This era saw an increased awareness of childhood as a blessed age of innocence, so cats became the accessory of choice in portraits of children, especially young girls". Bugler added: "And just as cats came increasingly to be seen as the natural companions for young children, so they gradually migrated into adult portraits of women, where their grace and mystery could complement the sensuality of the sitter" [52].

Two of the most famous English painters of this era—William Hogarth and Thomas Gainsborough—painted children with cats. Hogarth included a cat in his 1742 painting of "The Graham Children". He also included a cat standing next to a prostitute in his painting of "A Harlot's Progress". Gainsborough's 1781 painting of "Miss Brummell" suggested that cats were appropriate companions for young girls. He also painted "The Artists Daughter's With a Cat" and "Six Sketches of Cats." Paintings of children with cats had been rare in seventeenth-century English art but became much more common in the eighteenth century. Cats became the rightful playthings of young girls, as illustrated in Joseph Wright's 1770 painting of "Two Girls Dressing a Kitten by Candlelight". In other paintings, such as Johann Zoffrey's 1780 "Portrait of Sophia Dumergue," the daughter of an eminent London surgeon, the cat appears to emphasize her femininity (Fig. 4.2).

Given the increasing association of cats with children, it is not surprising that it was at this time that "Puss in Boots" appeared as a children's story. It is a fairy tale about how a cat used trickery to help his penniless master win the hand of a princess and live happily ever after. The story was translated from French into English in 1729, and the original edition depicted an old woman telling the story to a group of children with a placard inscribed "Mother Goose's Tales". The story was then adapted in 1812 by the Brothers Grimm, thereby confirming cats as respectable playthings for children.

Several prominent people in England's intellectual and arts community kept cats as pets in the eighteenth century. John Rich, an actor and theater manager who opened theaters at Lincoln Inn Fields in 1714 and Covent Garden in 1732, was said

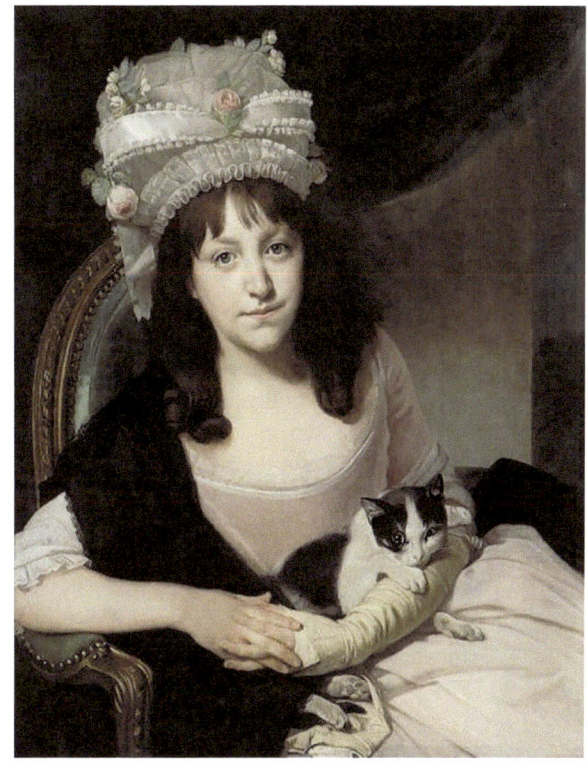

Fig. 4.2 Johann Zoffany, "Portrait of Sophie Dumergue", c. 1780. Oil on panel. The cat is apparently included to emphasize her femininity. Sophie was about 12 at the time. (Image courtesy of Victoria Art Gallery, Bath, under the Creative Commons License (CC BY-NC-ND))

to live with "7 and 20 cats of all sizes, colors, and kinds". Samuel Johnson, generally regarded as the leading English intellectual of the eighteenth century, owned many cats. Johnson's biographer, James Boswell, described Johnson's affection for his cats:

I never shall forget the indulgence with
which he treated Hodge, his cat; for whom he
himself used to go out and buy oysters, lest the
servants, having that trouble, should take a dislike
to the poor creature. I am, unluckily, one of those
who have an antipathy to a cat, so that I am uneasy
when in the room with one; and I own, I frequently
suffered a good deal from the presence of this same
Hodge. I recollect him one day scrambling up
Dr. Johnson's breast, apparently with much satisfaction,
while my friend smiling and half whistling, rubbed down
his back, and pulled him by the tail; and when I observed
he was a fine cat, saying "why yes, Sir, but I have had
cats whom I liked better than this," and then as if perceiving
Hodge to be out of countenance, adding, "but he is a
very fine cat, a very fine cat indeed".

In 1778 Hodge was immortalized by poet Percival Stockdale in "An Elegy on the Death of Dr. Johnson's Favourite Cat". Today a statue of Hodge sits outside the house where Samuel Johnson lived in London, and the cat has its own entry on Wikipedia [53, 54].

William Stukely was another intellectual of this period who enjoyed cats. Physician, clergyman, and archeologist, Stukely was a fellow of the Royal Society and pioneered the archeological investigations of Stonehenge and Avebury. In 1745 he memorialized his cat, noting that it had given him "much pleasure, without trouble" and relating the cat's "inimitable ways of testifying her love to her master and mistress". Essayist and politician Sir Richard Steele also liked cats; in an essay in *The Tatler*, he described the narrator coming home to his little dog and cat who welcome him "each of 'em in his proper Language" [55].

Horace Walpole was another leading eighteenth-century intellectual who was very fond of cats. The son of a British prime minister, Walpole was a novelist, prominent letter writer, and member of parliament. He owned at least two cats, one of which was immortalized in 1747 by the poet Thomas Gray. Gray, who was Walpole's closet friend and known as "the most learned man in Europe," wrote the poem for Walpole after one of his cats drowned in a large china tub filled with goldfish. In a letter accompanying the poem, Gray conveyed his own considerable affection for cats. The poem, titled "Ode on the Death of a Favourite Cat Drowned in a Tub of Goldfishes," opened with the cat sitting at the edge of the tub gazing wistfully at the fish. The oft-quoted denouement was inevitable:

Presumptuous maid! with looks intent
Again she stretch'd, again she bent,
Nor knew the gulf between.
(Malignant Fate sat by, and smiled)
The slippery verge her feet beguiled,
She tumbled headlong in.
Eight times emerging from the flood
She mewed to every watery god,
Some speedy aid to send.
No dolphin came, no Nereid stirred;
Nor cruel Tom, nor Susan heard;
A Favourite has no friend!
From hence, ye beauties, undeceived,
Know, one false step is ne'er retrieved,
And be with caution bold.
Not all that tempts your wandering eyes
And heedless hearts, is lawful prize;
Nor all that glisters, gold [56, 57].

Eighteenth century poets seemed to be inordinately attracted to cats, leading the French art critic who wrote under the name Champfleury to later claim that to understand cats "one must be a woman or a poet". In addition to Thomas Gray, two other prominent poets of this era who wrote poems about cats were Christopher Smart and William Cowper. Both men also suffered from periods of severe madness [58].

Christopher Smart, born in 1722, was initially regarded as one of the most promising poets of his generation. At Cambridge he was named the "scholar of the university" and later taught philosophy and rhetoric there. Moving to London, he went to work for the publisher Thomas Newberry and married Newberry's stepdaughter. His early poetry was well regarded by Samuel Johnson and others and won the Cambridge Seaton poetry prize five times in 6 years. The two poems for which Smart is best known are "A Song to David" and "Jubilate Agno"; the latter was incorporated into a cantata by composer Benjamin Britten.

It was during a period of psychiatric hospitalization that Smart wrote both of these poems. "Jubilate Agno" includes sections reflecting frankly psychotic thinking, including a "fascination with alphabetic sequence puns, word plays, sheer sound, and its relentless reiteration". Among cat lovers the best-known part of the poem is a long passage in which Smart praises his cat, Jeoffry:

> For I will consider my Cat Jeoffry.
> For he is the servant of the Living God duly and daily serving him.
> For at the first glance of the glory of God in the East he worships in his way.
> For this is done by wreathing his body seven times round with elegant quickness. For then he leaps up to catch the musk, which is the blessing of God upon his prayer.

Smart even claimed that his cat stood in opposition to the Devil, a surprising claim in an era when cats were still being persecuted because of their association with dark powers.

> For when his day's work is done his business more properly begins.
> For he keeps the Lord's watch in the night against the adversary.
> For he counteracts the powers of darkness by his electrical skin and glaring eyes.
> For he counteracts the Devil, who is death, by brisking about the life.
> For in his morning orisons he loves the sun and the sun loves him.
> For he is of the tribe of Tiger [57].

William Cowper, born in 1731, was said to have been "one of the most eminent poets of his time". William Wordsworth regarded Cowper as "the only poet whom he thought worthwhile learning off-by-heart". Cowper was especially fond of animals, including cats, and at one time was said to have also kept "two dogs, two goldfinches, two canaries, five rabbits, three hares, two guinea pigs, a squirrel, a magpie, a jay, and a starling". He was also a prolific letter writer, often including "his adventures with Puss" [59–62].

Among Cowper's better-known poems are two about cats. In "The Retired Cat," he described his cat as "A Poet's cat, sedate and grave/as poet well could wish to have," which goes to sleep in a partially open drawer in the poet's bedroom but then the housekeeper, not seeing the cat, shuts the drawer. That night Cowper was awakened when the cat made itself known. "The Colubriad," by contrast, described three of Cowper's kittens which were confronted by a viper snake:

> Close by the threshold of a door nailed fast
> Three kittens sat; each kitten looked aghast;
> I passing swift and inattentive by,

At the three kittens cast a careless eye,
Not much concerned to know what they did there,
Not deeming kittens worth a poet's care.
But presently a loud and furious hiss
Caused me to stop and to exclaim, 'What's this?'
When lo! upon the threshold met my view,
With head erect, and eyes of fiery hue,
A viper, long as Count de Grasse's queue.
Forth from his head his forked tongue he throws,
Darting it full against a kitten's nose,
Who having never seen, in field or house,
The like, sat still and silent as a mouse;
Only projecting with attention due,
Her whiskered face, she asked him, 'Who are you?'

Cowper then seized a garden hoe and summarily dispatched the snake [57].

4.9   Hospitals for Mad Persons

At the same time as cats were becoming established as common companions for artists, writers, and other intellectuals in eighteenth-century England, madness was becoming established as an increasing problem. The beds in Bethlem Hospital were continually full despite efforts by the hospital to restrict admissions to only those most in need. In a *Survey of the Cities of London and Westminster*, published in 1720, John Strype noted that "those are judged the fittest Objects for this Hospital [Bethlem] that are raving and furious and…likely to do mischief to themselves or others". Specifically excluded from admission were "those that are only Melancholik…or Ideots…these the Governores think the House [Bethlem] ought not be bothered with". Similarly, in *The History of Bethlem*, Jonathan Andrews claimed that "Bethlem was primarily a place for keeping lunatics who were a menace to themselves or others". A study of patients admitted to Bethlem Hospital between 1772 and 1787 reported that "above one half of the patients…have attempted some mischief against themselves or others…There are above a score of atrocious murderers: there are parricides, and butchers of their own offspring". By the 1780s there were 200 patients on the waiting list for admission. For readmissions, "Nearly two-thirds were forced to wait between five and nine years for the time their petitions were read before they were readmitted" [63–67].

As pressure for admission to Bethlem's limited number of beds increased, other psychiatric hospitals, both public and private, were being built. In Norwich, one of the largest cities outside of London, Mary Chapman left funds upon her death in 1724 to endow a public hospital for "distrest lunatiks". Chapman, the daughter of one of the city's wealthiest men, had had "lunacy…afflict some of my nearest relations and kindred" and founded the hospital "as a monument of my thankfulness to God" for having "blessed me with the free use of my reason and understanding". In 1725 London bookseller and member of parliament Thomas Guy left funds in his will to create a "lunatic house" in what would be called Guy's Hospital. In 1751

London's St. Luke's Hospital was opened by public subscription; a pamphlet entitled "Reasons for Establishing St. Luke's" noted Bethlem Hospital's overcrowding and long waiting list. In its first 10 years, St. Luke's admitted 749 patients, and by 1800 it had 300 beds, surpassing Bethlem in size. Additional psychiatric hospitals using public subscriptions were opened in 1764 in Newcastle, in 1766 in Manchester, in 1777 in York, in 1795 in Liverpool, and in 1801 in Oxford. Most of these facilities were small, with accommodations for 30 or fewer patients, but they represented a beginning for the increasing number of mentally ill individuals who were considered in need of hospitalization [68, 69].

It is noteworthy that subscribers who contributed funds for these hospitals did so specifically in response to perceived needs: for example, the founders of the Manchester Lunatic Hospital voted to raise the necessary funds for the hospital in order to provide care for "the Number of distressed Objects of this kind, with which this Kingdom unhappily abounds…no Cases could be more truly deplorable than those of Poor Lunatiks, who had in common no Prospect of a Cure and who…continued public Spectacles of the deepest Misery, if not Terror, to the Neighbors". Similarly, the Yorkshire Asylum was opened because of a belief that "something should be done for the relief of those unhappy sufferers who are the objects of terror and compassion to all around them and whose cases lay a just claim to the benevolence of their fellow creatures". According to Nigel Walker and Sarah McCabe, "an unmistakable phenomenon of this period was a growing public awareness of the special nature of the social problem posed by the mentally disordered," which showed itself "in the foundation by voluntary subscription of hospitals for the insane". Also representative of this growing public awareness was a sermon preached at St. Bridget's Church in London during Easter Week of 1759: "The Care of the Incurable Lunaticks, and the Charity Due to Them, Particularly Recommended" [70–73].

As the public psychiatric hospitals became more overcrowded in the eighteenth century, they increasingly restricted admission to the sickest and poorest patients. It thus became difficult for mentally ill individuals from upper class families to gain admission to the public hospitals, yet it was precisely the upper class that was apparently experiencing the fastest increase in madness and other nervous disorders. In response to this need for more upper-class beds, private madhouses proliferated. A few such facilities had opened in the closing years of the seventeenth century, especially in London, but during the first half of the eighteenth century, they increased rapidly in number. The problem was that there was no registration or regulation of them. Anyone could open a private madhouse, and it could be very profitable, so private madhouses were widely referred to as the trade in lunacy. Some of the private madhouses were run by respected physicians, such as William Battie who worked at the public St. Luke's Hospital as well as his own private facility, John Monro who worked at Bethlem Hospital as well as his own private facility; and Nathaniel Cotton who also wrote poetry and whose "Collegium Insanoraum" housed the poet Christopher Smart among others.

However, other private madhouses were run by individuals with no psychiatric skills, and the system was ripe for abuse. Wrongful confinement of sane persons in private madhouses was thematically used in several novels of the period, including Samuel Richardson's *Pamela; or Virtue Rewarded* (1740) and *Clarissa Harlowe* (1748), Tobias Smollett's *The Life and Adventures of Sir Launcelot Greaves* (1760), and Mary Wollstonecraft's *Maria* (1798). Several individuals who believed they had been wrongfully confined also published personal accounts, including Alexander Cruden (*The Adventures of Alexander the Corrector*, 1754) and Samuel Bruckshaw (*The Case, Petition and Address of Samuel Bruckshaw*, 1774). Both of these accounts include suggestions that the writers were indeed legitimately insane at the time of their involuntary confinement, despite their protestations to the contrary.

How often such private madhouse abuses actually happened in the eighteenth century is less clear. Patricia Allderidge suggested that "such cases were not frequent but were well publicized". William Parry-Jones, author of the definitive book on *The Trade in Lunacy*, also concluded that "despite the view that such abuses were widespread, surviving evidence for this is limited and often is based upon sensational accounts by persons of doubtful reliability". Finally in 1774, following parliamentary hearings, the Madhouses Act was passed establishing the licensing and inspection of all madhouses in London and vicinity [74, 75].

4.10 Public Interest in Madness

Perhaps the strongest evidence that madness was becoming more common in eighteenth-century England was the continuing intense public interest in the subject. In Cecil Moore's *Backgrounds of English Literature* 1700–1760, the author noted that "the seriousness of public interest [in mental disorders] is best reflected in letters, diaries, and other private records not intended for publication". Fiction of the period abounds with mad characters, beginning with Jonathan Swift's "Digression on Madness" in his 1704 *A Tale of a Tub*. English professor Michael DePorte claimed that "few writers of the eighteenth century were so morbidly fascinated by madness and madhouses as Swift". Regarding his satires, "madness is their obsessive theme; they expose and isolate one source of insanity after another and taken together they contain an alarming gallery of lunatics" [76, 77].

The theme of madness in literature continued throughout the century. The opening of Alexander Pope's narrative poem *The Dunciad* (1728) is set next to the walls of Bethlem. In Henry Fielding's *The Intriguing Chambermaid* (1733), Mr. Goodall is told that he is "a poor distracted wretch, and ought to have an apartment in a dark room, and clean straw". In Tobias Smollett's *Count Fathom* (1753), Elinor becomes insane and is sent to Bethlem Hospital to recover. In Laurence Sterne's *Tristam Shandy* (1760), Maria is also insane; the book was so popular that "Maria had inspired more than 30 paintings by the start of Victoria's reign". In Frances Sheridan's *Memoirs of Miss Sidney Biddulph* (1767), the protagonist is driven insane by guilt and confined to an asylum for the remainder of his life [78].

Visits to Bethlem, which had begun in the seventeenth century, intensified in the eighteenth. It was as if the public could not get enough of madness. English essayist Richard Steele took his three younger brothers "to show 'em ... Bedlam" and later sarcastically wrote that he had consulted "the collegiates of Moorfield," the part of London where Bethlem Hospital was located. Nicholas Blundell, visiting from Lancashire in 1703, "walked to Bedlam [sic]" and on two subsequent visits to London returned to the hospital to show his wife and daughters. Bethlem was a major attraction for foreign visitors as well. Travel guides such *as Les Delices de l'Angleterre* (1707) and *Travels in London* (1710) listed Bethlem as a major attraction. A German traveler at this time was intrigued by a patient "who is said to have crowed all day long like a cock" [79].

By the 1730s, the crowds at Bethlem included England's foremost aristocrats. The prince of Wales visited in 1735, the same year in which William Hogarth painted the eighth and final scene of *The Rake's Progress* on a Bethlem ward, showing an insane Thomas Rakewell being looked down upon by two noble ladies. In 1741 Samuel Richardson published *Familiar Letters on Important Occasions*, intended to provide "the requisite style and forms" for "letters written to and for particular friends on the most important occasions." One of his model letters was "from a young Lady in Town to her Aunt in the Country Describing Bethlem Hospital": "I have this afternoon been with my cousins to gratify the odd curiosity most people have to see Bethleham [sic] or Bedlam Hospital. A more affecting scene my eyes never beheld .... For there we see man destitute of every mark of reason and wisdom, and levell'd to the brute creation, if not beneath it" [80, 81].

By 1742 the flow of visitors to Bethlem had become a constant stream. The hospital governing board estimated that "about 19 thousand visitors" came each year to observe the approximately two hundred patients. That same year, the hospital governing board decided to appoint the hospital porter as a constable "to prevent disturbances ...at Holiday times." The crowds continued to increase and included such individuals as a young lady in 1752 who came "down from the country" to "see the tower, the [Westminster] abbey, and Bedlam, and two or three plays". By 1764 it became necessary to assign "four constables and also four stout fellows as assistants in each gallery" because "great riots and disorders have been committed in this hospital during the holidays." Because of the continuing disorder, 2 years later Bethlem Hospital was closed to all visitors on major holidays, and in 1770 it was closed to all visitors except those who had a ticket signed by the hospital's governor [82, 83].

The interest in viewing the insane in eighteenth-century England was quite extraordinary. A few visitors came out of "a moral duty, painful and distressing, yet pointing useful lessons .... A sight of Bethlem might be recommended as a peculiarly effective deterrent to the wayward inclinations of children". Most visitors, however, came to see the patients as "curiosities," "remarkable characters," and "very amusing objects". It was the titillation of a freak show, of viewing exotic human specimens not previously seen. Bethlem Hospital was thus regarded as a kind of human zoo, reminiscent of public exhibitions of lions, elephants, and other exotic creatures put on display by English explorers as they returned from Africa and Asia. In Henry Mackenzie's 1771 novel *The Man of Feeling*, Harley, the protagonist, described a visit to Bethlem Hospital, made because it was one of "those things called Sights in London, which every stranger is supposed desirous to see."

During the visit the hospital guide told Harley, "in the phrase of those that keep wild beasts for show," that patients in one particular ward "were much better worth seeing than any they had passed, being ten times more fierce and unmanageable." [84, 85]

4.11   Mad Poets

One of the characteristics of madness in eighteenth-century England was that it appeared to affect the upper social classes, and especially writers and intellectuals, disproportionately. This is best illustrated by Kay Jamison's study of 36 poets in her book *Touched with Fire*. All 36 of the poets were born between 1705 and 1805 and were selected because they were prominent in "15 anthologies of eighteenth- and nineteenth-century verse". Jamison then assessed their biographical information to ascertain how many were mentally ill. Among the 36 poets, she reported that 11 either had psychotic thinking, were confined to a psychiatric hospital, or committed suicide. She added that four others appear to have had bipolar disorder but not psychotic thinking or hospitalization. Altogether it would appear that at least one third of these poets would have been thought of as mad in the eighteenth century. And Jamison's list is not necessarily complete; it did not include Sir Charles Hanbury Williams, born in 1708, who was known as "the mad poet". As George S. Rousseau noted in 1969, "it is an ironic contrast that the supposed 'Age of Reason' should have produced so many cases of insanity among its writers" [86–88].

Christopher Smart, discussed above, was one example cited by Jamison. His psychiatric problems began in his 30s and focused on what was then called religious mania. He would suddenly drop to his knees in the middle of busy streets and insist that everyone around him join him in prayer. After several episodes of such behavior, punctuated by periods of depression, Smart was committed to newly opened St. Luke's Hospital for Lunatics where he remained for a year. Discharged as incurable, he then spent 4 more years in a private madhouse at Bethnal Green in London.

William Cowper was plagued by intermittent bouts of madness. These included auditory hallucinations, delusions that he had been dammed by God, a belief that other people could hear his thoughts, and severe depression. Cowper unsuccessfully tried on several occasions to take his own life by poison, drowning, stabbing, and hanging, and there are suggestions that he also castrated himself. He was hospitalized multiple times, including spending almost 2 years at Nathaniel Cotton's private madhouse at St. Albans. Cowper was acutely aware of his own madness and found it very unpleasant. He noted: "This of all maladies that man infect/Claims most compassion, and receives the least". And in a poem titled "Lines Written During a Period of Insanity," he wrote:

Man disavows, and Deity disowns me:
Hell might afford my miseries a shelter;
Therefore hell keeps her every hungry mouths all
Bolted against me [89–92].

One of Cowper's best-known poems, "The Task," described the madness of "a serving maid" whose lover dies at sea:
She heard the doleful tiding of his death—
And never smiled again! And now she roams
The dreary waste...
She begs an idle pin of all she meets,
And hoards them in her sleeve, but needful food,
Though pressed with hunger oft, or comlier clothes,
Though pinched with cold, asks never. Kate is crazed.

According to Phillip Martin, Cowper's description of Kate "was responsible for the massive popularity enjoyed by poems depicting madwomen in the magazines and miscellanies of the 1790s". Cowper's crazy Kate was also the inspiration for the numerous paintings, most notably Henry Fuseli's 1807 painting by that name, which was widely imitated. As Helen Small recently noted, "Between 1770 and about 1810, stories about bereaved or deserted women fallen into insanity were the subject of an extraordinary vogue in sentimental prose, poetry, drama, and painting" [93, 94].

In addition to Christopher Smart and William Cowper, William Collins was another mad poet cited by Jamison. He was born in 1721, educated at Oxford, and published his first poems at age 18. He then moved to London where he met Samuel Johnson. In his *Lives of the Most Eminent English Poets* (1779–1781), Johnson described Collins's work as follows: "He loved fairies, genii, giants, and monsters; he delighted to rove through the meanders of enchantment, to gaze on the magnificence of golden palaces, to repose by the water-falls of Elysian gardens". At age 32, Collins was "confined in a house of lunatics" because of "that depression of mind which enchains the faculties without destroying them, and leaves reason the knowledge of right without the power of pursuing it". Johnson also noted that Collins "puts his words out of the common order, seeming to think, with some later candidates for fame, that not to write prose is certainly to write poetry". Following discharge from the madhouse, Collins lived with his sister and died at age 38 [95].

Thomas Chatterton, born in 1752, was said by Jamison to have had bipolar disorder. Regarded as one of England's most brilliant young poets, Chatterton published his first poems at age 11. At 15 he began publishing poems that he attributed to the lost writings of a fictitious fifteenth-century monk named Thomas Rowley. The poems were well regarded, and Chatterton maintained his hoax for a year until he was finally unmasked by Horace Walpole. A year later, at age 17, Chatterton killed himself by swallowing arsenic and became "an emblem for the English romantic movement". Samuel Taylor Coleridge published a "Monody on the Death of Chatterton". John Keats dedicated a poem to Chatterton, "the Most English of Poets except Shakespeare". And William Wordsworth would remember him as "the marvelous Boy, the Sleepless South that perished in his pride" [96].

At the time Chatterton took his life, suicide was on the increase in England and widely regarded as a form of madness. An article in a popular journal in 1720 claimed that "more people kill themselves in this one country [England] than in the rest of the entire world combined". In 1737 a French visitor to London was quoted as being astonished "to hear of such frequent self-murders [sic] as happens here almost daily". In 1743 Scottish poet Robert Blair published "The Grave" which included these lines:

Self-murder!—name it not: Our island's shame,
That makes her the reproach of neighboring states [97].

Thomas Gray was another poet who claimed that suicide in England had become "epidemical". Gray himself suffered from what he called "white Melancholy…which though it seldom laughs or dances…is a good easy sort of state". However, it sometimes became black melancholy which "excludes and shuts its eyes to the most possible hopes, and everything that is pleasurable". In two lines in his poem "Ode on a Distant Prospect of Eton College," Gray eloquently captured the contradictory feelings inherent in his melancholy:

And moody Madness laughing wild
Amid severest woe [98, 99].

4.12 The English Malady

In 1733 George Cheyne, a prominent London physician, published a widely read book titled *The English Malady*. Cheyne had been stimulated to write the book by his concern about suicide. He had become alarmed by the "late Frequency and daily Encrease of wanton and uncommon self-murderers, produc'd mostly by this Distemper". Cheyne focused much attention on "spleen, vapors, lowness of spirits, and hypochondriacal and hysterical distempers" which he regarded as being the less severe end of the spectrum of distempers, with "true Manias, real Lunacy [and] Madness" on the more severe end. The less severe nervous disorders were merely "a lower Degree of Lunacy, and the first Step towards a distemper'd Brain" [100, 101].

Cheyne believed that nervous disorders were especially common in England:

The Title I have chosen for this Treatise, is a Reproach universally thrown on this island by Foreigners, and all our Neighbours on the Continent, by whom nervous Distempers, Spleen, Vapours, and Lowness of Spirits', are in Derision, called the ENGLISH MALADY. And I wish there were not so good Grounds for this Reflection.

He also believed that such disorders were increasing in frequency and severity. "They were scarce known to our Ancestors, and never rising to such fatal Heights, nor afflicting such Numbers in any other known Nation". "In England alone..I have been told that a late worthy and learned Physician, that had examin'd into the Numbers confin'd for Lunacy and Madness, upon the strictest Examination, found they reach'd to a Number I dare not name". Another aspect of the nervous disorders that impressed Cheyne was that they seemed to occur most commonly among people "of the better sort". By "better sort" Cheyne meant that such disorders "seldom and I think never happens or can happen, to any but those of the liveliest and quickest natural Parts, whose Faculties are the brightest and most spiritual, and whose Genius is most keen and penetrating, and particularly where there is the most delicate Sensation and Taste, both of Pleasure and Pain" [102].

As one of the best-known London physicians of his era, Cheyne counted among his patients David Hume, John Wesley, Alexander Pope, and Samuel Johnson. Johnson was impressed by Cheyne and by *The English Malady*, and he recommended the book to James Boswell. Johnson had an intense interest in nervous disorders because of his own problems, a mixture of symptoms that today would be diagnosed as obsessive-compulsive disorder and Tourette's syndrome. For example, he regularly touched every post along the street as he walked, avoided stepping on the paving stones, and, according to Boswell, exited doorways "by a certain number of steps from a certain point, or at least so that either his right or his left foot…should constantly make the first actual movement when he came close to the door or passage". Johnson was intensely troubled by his obsessions and compulsions, believing they were a sign of impending madness. Such was his fear of going completely mad that, "as a precautionary measure, [Johnson] apparently entrusted his great friend, Mrs. Hester Thrale, with a chain and padlock, for emergency use" [103–105].

A shared interest in madness was a strong bond between Johnson and Boswell, his friend and eventual biographer. Both men had experienced periods of serious depression. Both men had visited Bethlem to observe mad people—Johnson apparently on more than one occasion and Boswell in 1771. Both men wrote about madness. Johnson did so in his 1759 *Rasselas* in which an astronomer becomes delusional and believes he can control the sun; Boswell did so in a series of essays he published in the *London Magazine* between 1777 and 1783 under the title "The Hypochodriack." Where Johnson and Boswell differed was on the relationship between madness and lesser forms of nervous disorders. Johnson, like George Cheyne, believed that the conditions were on a spectrum with madness simply being a more severe variant of melancholy or other nervous disorders. Thus Johnson was perpetually afraid that his own depression or obsessive-compulsive symptoms would slide down the spectrum into madness. Boswell, by contrast, believed that madness was fundamentally different from the other disorders. As described by him, "Dr. Johnson and I had a serious conversation by ourselves on melancholy and madness: which he was, I always thought, enormously inclined to confound together. Melancholy, like 'great wit' may be near allied to madness; but there is, in my opinion, a distinct separation between them". Boswell himself knew the difference, since "one of his own children, Euphenia, was mentally deranged," and his brother, John, was intermittently insane and confined in private asylums. On one occasion Boswell reflected on his brother's illness: "It was a curious sensation when I saw my brother, with whom I had been brought up, in such a state. Madness of every degree is inexplicable" [106, 107].

When Samuel Johnson published *Rasselas* in 1759, one of his characters noted: "Of all the uncertainties of our present state, the most dreadful and alarming is the uncertain continuance of reason". In fact, Johnson believed that madness was increasing in prevalence and told Boswell that it had "grown more frequent since smoking had gone out of fashion," since he thought smoking tranquilized the mind. In believing that madness was increasing, he was following the claim of Cheyne's *The English Malady* [108, 109].

As the eighteenth century progressed, others began to share Cheyne's concern. In 1735, 2 years after the publication of Cheyne's book, a letter to the Royal College of Physicians referred to madness as "epidemical" and noted: "Our nation has been observed by foreigners to abound in maniacs, more than any other upon the face of the earth…I find it has of late increased so much among us, that there is scarce a family in the nation entirely free from it". In 1750, the anonymous author of *A Treatise on the Dismal Effects of Low-Spiritedness* claimed that the problem was "almost peculiar to, and epidemical in, this kingdom". In 1758 William Battie, one of the most respected physicians in London and who had been on the board of governors for Bethlem, called madness "a terrible and at present very frequent calamity". In 1778 William Perfect, the owner of a private madhouse, published his book on *Select Cases in the Different Species of Insanity* in which he claimed that "instances of insanity are at this day more numerous in this kingdom than they were at any former period". Then in 1788 William Rowley published a book on nervous disorders in women and asserted that "England, according to its size and number of inhabitants, produces and contains more insane than any other country in Europe". In the closing years of the eighteenth century, books about psychiatric disorders in general and insanity in particular proliferated rapidly. According to one study, between 1701 and 1744, 24 such books were published in England, but from 1745 to 1788, an additional 64 such books were published [110–112].

And then the unimaginable happened. In November, 1788, King George III developed a fever and other physical symptoms. Over the next several weeks, his illness progressed to delusions, hallucinations, mania, and violent outbursts that required the use of restraints. At first the king's physicians said little publicly, but rumors circulated among the public, including a rumor that the king had died. Eventually, however, the true story came out—the king himself had become mad. Here, then, for many was a confirmation of the magnitude of the English malady.

References

1. Scarre G. Witchcraft and magic in 16th and 17th century Europe. London: Macmillan; 1987. p. 23.
2. Scarre G. Witchcraft and magic in 16th and 17th century Europe. London: Macmillan; 1987. See also the entries for James I and Daemonology on Wikipedia. Accessed 6 May, 2019. https://en.wikipedia.org/wiki/Daemonologie.
3. Mathew Hopkins entry on Wikipedia. https://en.wikipedia.org/wiki/Matthew_Hopkins.
4. Thomas K. Man and the natural world. New York, Oxford; 1983. p. 109–10.
5. Thomas K. Man and the natural world. New York, Oxford; 1983. p. 110, 118.
6. Thomas K. Man and the natural world. New York, Oxford; 1983. p. 112–6.
7. Thomas K. Man and the natural world. New York, Oxford; 1983. p. 102–4, 111.
8. Serpell J. In the company of animals. Oxford: Basil Blackwell; 1986. p. 40.
9. Thomas K. Man and the natural world. New York, Oxford; 1983. p. 111.
10. Zimmer C. Soul made flesh. New York: Free Press; 2004. p. 102.
11. Thomas K. Man and the natural world. New York, Oxford; 1983. p. 118.

12. Rogers KM. Cat. London: Reaktion Books: 2006. p. 82.
13. Tabor R. Cats: The rise of the cat. London, BCA; 1991. p. 58. This ratio coincides exactly with an informal survey I did at the Louvre in Paris of all paintings there dated prior to the 18th Century.
14. Bugler C. The Cat: 3,500 years of the cat in art. New York: Merrell; 2011. p. 204.
15. MacDonald M. Mystical bedlam, madness, anxiety and healing in seventeenth-century England. Cambridge, U.K.: Cambridge University Press; 1981. p. 2.
16. Dalby JT. Elizabethan madness: on London's stage. Psychol Rep. 1997; 81:1331–43.
17. Andrews J, et al. The History of Bethlem. London: Routledge; 1997. p. 130.
18. MacDonald M. Mystical bedlam, madness, anxiety and healing in seventeenth-century England. Cambridge, U.K.: Cambridge University Press; 1981. p. 122.
19. Collins J. Lunatics in literature. North American Review. 1923; 218:376–87.
20. Andrews J, et al. The History of Bethlem. London: Routledge; 1997. p. 132.
21. Reed RR. Bedlam on the Jacobean stage. Cambridge: Harvard University Press; 1952. p. 39.
22. Andrews J, et al. The History of Bethlem. London: Routledge; 1997. p. 167.
23. DePorte MV. Nightmares and hobby horses. San Marino: Huntington Library; 1974. p. 3.
24. Andrews J, et al. The History of Bethlem. London: Routledge; 1997. p. 51.
25. O'Donoghue E. The story of Bethlem Hospital. London: Unwin; 1914. p. 152.
26. Scull A. The most solitary of afflictions. New Haven: Yale University Press; 1993. p. 11.
27. Andrews J, et al. The History of Bethlem. London: Routledge; 1997. p. 187, 190.
28. Andrews J, et al. The History of Bethlem. London: Routledge; 1997. p. 233.
29. Leigh D. The historical development of British psychiatry, vol 1. Oxford: Pergamon; 1961. p. 3.
30. Andrews J, et al. The history of Bethlem. London: Routledge; 1997. p. 189–90, 178, 186.
31. Porter R, Manacles M-F. A history of madness in England. Cambridge: Harvard University Press; 1987. p. 126.
32. Porter R. A social history of madness. New York: Weidenfield and Nicolson; 1987. p. 62–3.
33. Andrews J, et al. The history of Bethlem. London: Routledge; 1997. p. 3–4.
34. Porter R. A social history of madness. New York: Weidenfield and Nicolson; 1987. p. 3.
35. DePorte MV. Nightmares and hobby horses. San Marino: Huntington Library; 1974. p. 108–9.
36. MacDonald M. The inner side of wisdom: suicide in early modern England. Psychol Med. 1977;7:565–82.
37. MacDonald M. Mystical bedlam, madness, anxiety and healing in seventeenth-century England. Cambridge, U.K.: Cambridge University Press; 1981. p. 112.
38. Byrd M. Visits to bedlam: madness and literature in the eighteenth century. Columbia: University of South Carolina Press; 1974. p. 116–7.
39. MacDonald M. Mystical bedlam, madness, anxiety and healing in seventeenth-century England. Cambridge, U.K.: Cambridge University Press; 1981. p. 3.
40. MacDonald M. Mystical bedlam, madness, anxiety and healing in seventeenth-century England. Cambridge, U.K.: Cambridge University Press; 1981. p. 11.
41. Porter R. Mind-forg'd manacles: The history of madness in England from the Restoration to the Regency. Cambridge; Harvard University Press: 1987. p.136.
42. Porter R. Mind-forg'd manacles: The history of madness in England from the Restoration to the Regency. Cambridge; Harvard University Press: 1987. p. 137.
43. Andrews J, et al. The history of Bethlem. London: Routledge; 1997. p. 203.
44. Porter R. Mind-forg'd manacles: The history of madness in England from the Restoration to the Regency. Cambridge; Harvard University Press: 1987. p. 138.
45. Thomas K. Man and the natural world. New York, Oxford; 1983. p. 110.
46. Mery F. The life, history and magic of the cat. London: Paul Hamlyn; 1967. p. 56.
47. Scull A. The most solitary of afflictions. New Haven: Yale University Press; 1993. p. 105.
48. Rogers KM. Cat. London: Reaktion Books: 2006. p. 62.
49. Jane Wenham entry on Wikipedia
50. Kete K. The beast in the boudoir. Berkeley: University of California Press; 1994. p. 123–44.
51. Tague IH. Animal companions: pets and social change in eighteenth-century Britain. University Park: Pennsylvania State University Press; 2015. p. 63.

52. Bugler C. The Cat: 3,500 years of the cat in art. New York: Merrell; 2011. p. 24–5, 201.
53. Tabor R. Cats: The rise of the cat. London, BCA; 1991. p. 58.
54. Boswell J. The life of Samuel Johnson, LLD. New York: Dell Publishing; 1960; originally published in 1791. p. 330.
55. Rogers KM. Cat. London: Reaktion Books: 2006. p. 84–5.
56. Sherburne G, Bond DF. The restoration and the eighteenth century—A literary history of England. London: Oxford; 1967. p. 1075.
57. https://www.poemhunter.com.
58. Kete K. The beast in the boudoir. Berkeley: University of California Press; 1994. p. 126.
59. John NM. The uses of madness: William Cowper's 'Memoir'. Am Scholar. 34(1964-65):112–26.
60. Ella GM. William Cowper: The man of God's stamp. Dundas, Ontario: Joshua Press; 2000. p. 110.
61. Winslow HM. Concerning cats. Boston: Lothrop Publishing; 1900. p. 164.
62. Sherburne G, Bond DF. The restoration and the eighteenth century—A literary history of England. London: Oxford; 1967. p. 1076.
63. Strype J. quoted in Andrews J. The lot of the 'incurably' insane in enlightenment England. Eighteenth-Century Life 12(1); 1988. p. 1–18.
64. Andrews J, et al. The history of Bethlem. London: Routledge; 1997. p. 126.
65. Hunter R, Macalpine I. Three hundred years of psychiatry. London: Oxford University Press; 1963. p. 645, quoting William Black's "A dissertation on insanity," 1788.
66. Andrews J, et al. The history of Bethlem. London: Routledge; 1997. p. 232.
67. Andrews J. The lot of the 'incurably' insane in enlightenment England. Eighteenth-Century Life 12(1); 1988.
68. Allderidge P. Hospitals, madhouses and asylums. Br J Psychiat. 1999;134:321–34.
69. Leigh D. The historical development of British psychiatry, vol 1. Oxford: Pergamon; 1961.
70. Anonymous, An account of the rise, and present establishment of the lunatick hospital, in Manchester. Manchester: J. Harrop; 1771.
71. Digby A. Madness, morality and medicine: a study of the York Retreat 1796–1914. Cambridge: Cambridge University Press; 1985. p. 11.
72. Walker N. McCabe S. Crime and insanity in England. Edinburgh: University Press; 1968. p. 70.
73. Hunter R, Macalpine I. Three hundred years of psychiatry. London: Oxford University Press; 1963. p. 419.
74. Allderidge P. Hospitals, madhouses and asylums. Br J Psychiat. 1999;134:321–34.
75. Parry-Jones W. The trade in lunacy: a study of the private madhouses in England in the eighteenth and nineteenth centuries. London: Routledge and Kegan Paul; 1972. p. 289.
76. Moore CA. Backgrounds of English literature. New York: Octagon Books; 1969. p. 200.
77. DePorte MV. Nightmares and hobby horses. San Marino: Huntington Library; 1974. p. 57–8.
78. Small H. Love's madness: medicine, the novel, and female insanity, 1800–1865.   Oxford: Clarendon Press; 1996. p 11-12. 13.
79. Andrews J, et al. The history of Bethlem. London: Routledge; 1997. p. 183–4, 6.
80. Andrews J, et al. The history of Bethlem. London: Routledge; 1997. p. 180.
81. Richardson S. Familiar letters on important occasions. Norwood, PA: Norwood Editions; 1975; first published in 1741. p. 201.
82. Webster on the study of mental diseases (review article on John Webster's observations on the admission of medical pupils to the wards of Bethlem Hospital, for the purpose of studying mental diseases). Monthly Rev. 1842;162(3):74–88.
83. Andrews J, et al. The history of Bethlem. London: Routledge; 1997. p. 186, 190.
84. Andrews J, et al. The history of Bethlem. London: Routledge; 1997. p. 183, 186.
85. Mackenzie H. The man of feeling, ch. 20. London: Oxford University Press; 1967; originally published in 1771.
86. Jamison KR. Touched with fire: manic-depressive illness and the artistic temperament. New York: Free Press; 1993. p. 292, 62-71.
87. Moore CA. Backgrounds of English literature. New York: Octagon Books; 1969. p. 231.

88. Rousseau GS. Science and the discovery of the imagination in enlightened England. Eighteenth-Century Stud. 1969;3:117.
89. Porter R. A social history of madness. New York: Weidenfield and Nicolson; 1987. p. 94.
90. Wright T. The life of William Cowper. London: Unwin; 1892.
91. Moore CA. Backgrounds of English literature. New York: Octagon Books; 1969. p. 191.
92. Ella GM. William Cowper: The man of God's stamp. Dundas, Ontario: Joshua Press; 2000. p. 156.
93. Martin PW. Mad women in romantic writing. New York: St. Martin's Press; 1987. p. 19.
94. Small H. Love's madness: medicine, the novel, and female insanity, 1800–1865. Oxford: Clarendon Press; 1996. p. 11–12.
95. Johnson S. Lives of the English poets. Oxford: Clarendon Press; 1905. p. 337–9.
96. Kaplan LJ. Thomas Chatterton. Berkeley: University of California Press; 1987. p. 1, 17.
97. Moore CA. Backgrounds of English literature. New York: Octagon Books; 1969. p. 201, 205.
98. Moore CA. Backgrounds of English literature. New York: Octagon Books; 1969. p. 207.
99. Porter R. Mind-forg'd manacles: The history of madness in England from the Restoration to the Regency. Cambridge; Harvard University Press: 1987. p. 94.
100. DePorte MV. Nightmares and hobby horses. San Marino: Huntington Library; 1974. p. 147.
101. Byrd M. Visits to bedlam: madness and literature in the eighteenth century. Columbia: University of South Carolina Press; 1974. p. 120–1.
102. Hunter R, Macalpine I. Three hundred years of psychiatry. London: Oxford University Press; 1963. p. 351–4.
103. Viets HR. George Cheyne, 1673-1743. Bulletin History Med. 1949;23:435–52.
104. Boswell J. The life of Samuel Johnson, LLD. New York: Dell Publishing; 1960; originally published in 1791. p. 130.
105. Porter R, editor. The Faber book of madness. London: Faber and Faber; 1991. p. 113.
106. Byrd M. Visits to bedlam: madness and literature in the eighteenth century. Columbia: University of South Carolina Press; 1974. p. 94.
107. Vulliamy CE, Boswell J. Freeport, N.Y.: Books for Libraries Press; 1932. p. 269; Ryskamp C, Pottle FA (eds.) Boswell, The ominous years, 1774–1776. New York: McGraw-Hill; 1963. p. 44.
108. Hunter R, Macalpine I. Three hundred years of psychiatry. London: Oxford University Press; 1963. p. 417.
109. Anonymous. Miscellany: Dr. Samuel Johnson on insanity. Am J Insanity. 1847;3:285–7.
110. Anonymous. An account of the progress of an epidemical madness. London: J. Roberts; 1735.
111. Moore CA. Backgrounds of English literature. New York: Octagon Books; 1969. p. 193–4.
112. Hunter R, Macalpine I. Three hundred years of psychiatry. London: Oxford University Press; 1963. p. 405.

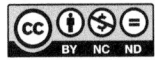

The Rise of Cats and Madness: III. The Nineteenth Century

5

5.1 The King's Madness

Nineteenth-century England saw a marked increase in both the status and the number of cats as pets. All classes of society welcomed cats to their households, and a picture of a cat by the fireside became an image for the ideal English home. During the same years, the number of insane persons in England increased dramatically. In 1829, the first reliable national census counted 8,941 insane persons or 0.79 per 1,000 population. In 1915 the census counted 140,461 insane persons or 3.98 per 1,000 population, a fivefold increase in 86 years.

The insanity of King George III shocked England and permanent1ly altered the way madness was viewed. As noted by British historians Ida Macalpine and Richard Hunter, "No longer could insanity be equated with ignorance or sin or superstition. If it was possible for the highest in the land to be struck down after an utterly blameless life of devotion to duty…surely such an illness could not be anything but natural, demanding of sympathy and amenable to medicine as any other?" [1]

The king recovered from his first episode of psychosis after 5 months, and the archbishop of Canterbury composed a prayer of thanksgiving. In retrospect, the cause of the king's insanity was almost certainly acute intermittent porphyria, a rare genetic disease with both physical and psychiatric symptoms. King George had additional attacks in 1801, 1804, and 1810 by which time he was largely blind, deaf, and senile, and he finally died in 1820.

It was during King George's reign that England laid the groundwork for becoming a nineteenth-century superpower. Lord Nelson defeated the Spanish fleet in 1797 and the French fleet the following year, thus ruling the seas. By the time of the king's death, England had colonized much of the West Indies, parts of Canada, Sierra Leone and Gambia in West Africa, Ceylon and parts of India, and Java. Despite the loss of its American colonies, the sun never set on the British Empire. The trade with its colonies, in turn, stimulated industrialization at home where cottage industries such as textile manufacturing moved to factories driven by water

© E. Fuller Torrey 2022
E. F. Torrey, *Parasites, Pussycats and Psychosis*,
https://doi.org/10.1007/978-3-030-86811-6_5

power and steam engines. As the nineteenth century advanced, England became the wealthiest country on earth.

One consequence of this increasing wealth was a rapidly expanding middle class with money to spare and aspirations for living like the upper class. One symbol of upper-class living was the keeping of pets, especially dogs. As noted by Ingrid Tague in *Animal Companions: Pets and Social Change in Eighteenth-Century Britain*, the English middle class had traditionally regarded pet-keeping as "a wasteful extravagance…at best a useless luxury, at worst it was actually sinful." However, "by 1800 attitudes had changed so much that many people had come to regard the love of pets as a sign of moral virtue rather than corruption." Hundreds of London street traders offered live animals, especially dogs, for sale. Books on dogs and products such as Spratts Patent Meat "Fibrine" Dog Cakes ("As supplied to the Royal Kennels") became available. As Harriet Ritvo noted in *The Animal Estate*, "by the middle of the nineteenth century what has been called the Victorian cult of pets was firmly established" [2, 3].

The cult of pet-keeping was called "Victorian" for good reason. Queen Victoria, the only child of the fourth son of King George III, ascended the throne in 1837 and proceeded to set new standards for royal pet-keeping. During her reign she had 88 pets, all named, including 2 Shetland ponies given to her by King Victor Emmanuel of Italy and 2 Tibetan goats, a present from the Shah of Persia. Most of her pets were dogs of various breeds, and she is said to have "had portraits painted of every one of her pampered canines" [4].

5.2   Nineteenth-Century Cats

Queen Victoria also kept a few cats, most notably a Persian named "White Heather." The fact that the queen kept cats would certainly have helped negate any lingering stigma associated with their diabolic past. In her book *Cat*, Katherine Rogers noted that "cats were widely appreciated as pets in the nineteenth century, but they did not contribute to their owners' prestige like dogs or horses." Others agree that at this time "cats were often classed with rabbits and cavies (guinea pigs) as lesser fancy animals and pets of the working man" [5–7]. Nevertheless, many well-known English people owned cats. Florence Nightingale, for example, owned more than 60 cats in her lifetime and claimed that they "possessed much more sympathy and feeling than human beings" [5–7].

Paintings from this period illustrate how the cat was viewed. Walter Crane, an English artist and illustrator of children's books, placed their family cat beside the fireplace in a portrait of his wife (Fig. 5.1). A book on life in the English countryside in the nineteenth century emphasized the importance of "the cat by the fireside or the canary singing in its cage" as symbols of "the comfort of the home." Katherine Rogers agreed that during the nineteenth century the cat became identified "with the Victorian ideal of Home…It became an embodiment of domestic virtue." For example, *The Happy Home*, a religious tract, was illustrated with a picture of a father

Fig. 5.1 Walter Crane, "At Home: A Portrait", 1872, Tempora on paper. A cat by the fireside became a symbol of an ideal British home. (Image courtesy of Leeds Museums and Galleries (Leeds Art Gallery) U.K. Copywrite: Leeds Museums and Galleries/ Bridgemen Images)

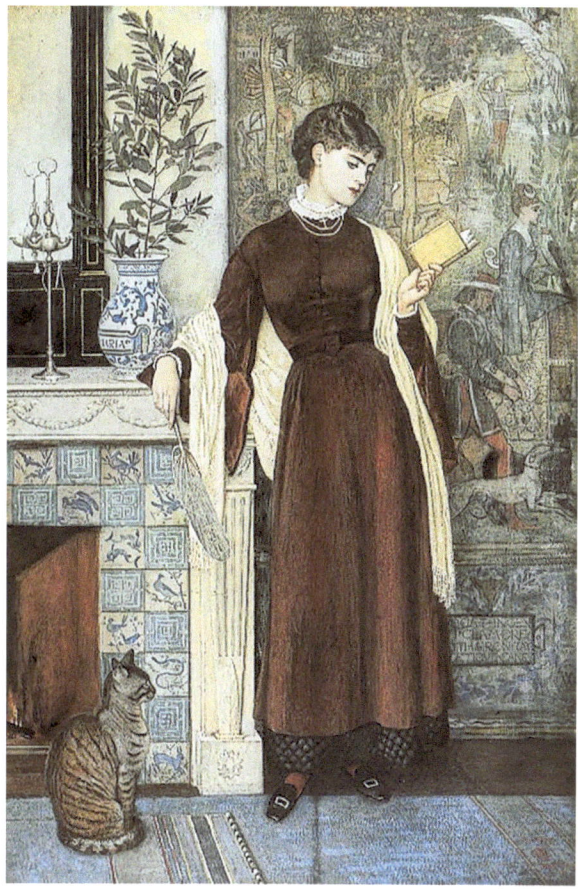

reading to his wife and four children with a cat standing in the foreground, "obviously also listening attentively" [8].

At this time cats were also increasingly associated with women, especially young women and female children. French painter Louis-Leopold Boilly painted a 2-year-old girl holding a cat. An 1835 article in a popular London magazine described children at play, "dressing themselves, or a favorite dog or kitten, in the most ludicrous and fanciful attire." Ford Madox Brown painted his daughter picking flowers with a cat at her feet. Another aspect of femininity was the association of cats with sexuality, as depicted by the French painter Edouard Manet in his 1862 portrait of "Olympia," a prostitute with a cat. In *Beastly Possessions*, Sarah Amato claims that at this time "grown men were not pictured with cats," which makes Sir John Everett Millais' 1850 portrait of a man holding a cat unusual [9, 10].

As had been true in the eighteenth century, writers and especially poets continued to be among the most enthusiastic cat lovers in the nineteenth century. Robert Southey, poet laureate of England from 1813 until his death in 1843, was an example. He kept many cats at his home at Keswick in the Lake Country, a home he shared with the family of Samuel Taylor Coleridge and which was regularly visited by Byron, Keats, Shelley, and Scott among others. Southey's son later wrote how his father enjoyed naming his cats:

> He rejoiced in bestowing upon them the strangest appellations; and it was not a little amusing to see a kitten answer to the name of some Italian singer or Indian chief, or hero of a German fairy tale, and often names and titles were heaped one upon another, til the possessor, unconscious of the honour conveyed, used to 'set up his eyes and look' in wonderment.

When one of his favorite cats died, Southey wrote to his friend Grosvenor Bedford who was a fellow lover of cats:

> Alas, Grosvenor, this day poor Rumpel was found dead, after a long and happy a life as cat could wish for, if cats form wishes on that subject. His full titles were: The Most Noble, the Archduke Rumpelstilszchen, Marcus Macbum, Earl Tomlefnagne, Baron Raticide, Waowhler and Scratch. There should be a court-mourning in Catland, and if the Dragon (your pet cat) wear a black ribbon around his neck, or a band of crape *a la militaire* round one of his fore paws it will be but a becoming mark of respect...I believe we are each and all, servants included, more sorry for his loss, or rather more affected by it, than any one of us would like to confess [11, 12].

John Keats wrote a "Sonnet To A Cat" as well as a tribute to the aging cat of a friend: "To Mrs Reynold's Cat." Percy Bysshe Shelley's first known poem was "Verses On a Cat," and he was once quoted as saying: "When my cats aren't happy, I'm not happy. Not because I care about their mood, but because I know they are just sitting there, thinking up ways to get even." George Gordon, Lord Byron, owned five cats at one time along with eight dogs, three monkeys, and a pet bear [13, 14].

Sir Walter Scott was said to have "loved all his pets and particularly pampered his cats," especially his favorite named "Hinx." He wrote to a friend: "Ah! Cats are a mysterious kind of folk. There is more passing in their minds then we are aware of. It comes no doubt from their being too familiar with warlocks and witches." William Wordsworth wrote a poem "See The Kitten on the Wall" and was quoted as saying that a kitten "is infinitely more amusing than half the people one is obliged to live with in this world." Algernon Swinburne was said to be "devoted to cats," especially his favorite named "Atossa," and wrote a poem, "To a Cat." John Clare, whose poetry celebrated the English countryside, included cats in several of his poems, including one titled "The Cat Runs Races with Her Tail" [15, 16].

A biographer of William Blake noted that "Blake always preferred cats to dogs." Blake, who was an artist as well as a poet, painted six watercolors to illustrate Thomas Gray's "Ode On the Death of a Favorite Cat," a poem about the drowning of Horace Walpole's cat. Charles Dickens owned several cats, including William which was obligingly renamed Williamina after it gave birth to kittens. When his cat named Bob died, Dickens had one paw stuffed and used it as a letter opener. He was quoted as saying: "What greater gift than the love of a cat." Although he personally liked cats, they are said to be "menacing in his novels." In *Bleak House*, for example, the large gray cat "is deeply disquieting as she...slinks reluctantly from a dead man's room…She embodies the predacity that Dickens saw throughout his society" [17].

The Bronte sisters were also known as cat lovers. In 1842 Emily wrote an essay on "The Cat" in which she noted: "I can say with sincerity that I like cats, also I can give you very good reasons why those who despise them are wrong." According to Katherine Rogers, Anne and Charlotte Bronte "introduced cats into their novels to mark the difference between sensitive people, who consider the feelings of an animal regardless of its conventional status, and obtuse ones, who despise cats as the associates of women and peasants" [18].

It should be noted that England was not unique in the attraction of its writers and other artists to cats. Katherine Rogers claimed that "it would be hard to find a major nineteenth-century French writer who was not particularly fond of cats." These included poets Charles Baudelaire, Thèophile Gautier, and Stephane Mallarme and the historian and critic Hippolyte Taine. Taine described himself as the "friend, master, and servant" of three cats, and he dedicated 12 sonnets to them. He also was quoted as saying: "I have studied many philosophers and many cats. The wisdom of cats is infinitely superior." Rogers noted that "cats with their traditional demonic associations were a perfect symbol for the artist's rejection of conventional standards and assumptions… A taste for what is demonic and forbidden, in cat as in artist, indicated superiority because it proved one's ability to see through the obtuse complacency of ordinary people" [19, 20].

Thus, by the latter half of the nineteenth century, cats had become respectable as pets. It was not only eccentric ladies who favored cats, such as "Mrs. Greggs of London who bequeathed 150 pounds per annum so that a trusted black servant could continue to care for her 86 cats." Cats had been lauded by prominent intellectuals such as Samuel Johnson, leading poets such as Robert Southey, and popular novelists such as Charles Dickens and the Bronte sisters. Whereas cats had once been burned as representations of Satan, they had risen from the ashes and assumed a proud place beside the fireplace as representatives of a proper English home [21].

Perhaps nothing symbolized the achievement of feline respectability more than the first English cat show. It took place at London's Crystal Palace on July 16, 1871, organized by Harrison Weir, an artist who was interested in different cat breeds. There were 160 caged entries, with Weir and his brother acting as judges. The cat show was not only the first such show to be held in England but probably in the world. It marked a new relationship between cats and humans. The cat show became an annual event in London and several other English cities and led to the chartering of a national cat club in 1887 with "many well-known people as members, life members, or associates." One of the main purposes of the club was to keep a national studbook and register "in which are registered pedigrees and championship wins" from the cat shows. Thus, each registered cat, which was given a unique number for one shilling per cat, was listed by its sire and dam as well as by its owner. By 1900 there was said to be 2000 registered cats in the studbook, one of which was "valued at 3500 pounds sterling—as much as the price of a first-class race horse." *Felis silvestris*, which had begun hanging around early agricultural settlements 10,000 years earlier, had truly arrived socially by the late nineteenth century when people started keeping records of its parentage. The cat had become not merely respectable but also respected [22].

By the close of the nineteenth century, cats had become increasingly popular as pets. One contemporary source estimated 350,000 cats for all of England; another estimated 400,000 of which half were said to be "unattached," for London alone. And they were popular: "It is certain that they [cats] have more really friends there than in any other country... Queen Victoria and the Princess of Wales, and indeed many members of the nobility are cat lovers, and doubtless this fact influences the general sentiment in England." The keeping of cats and other pets was no longer confined to the upper or even middle classes; "even very poor families between 1870 and 1914 participated in these new consumption patterns...[including] the ownership of pets" [23–27].

One measure of the increasing popularity of cats at this time was the increased use of them in advertisements to sell products. According to a history of cats, "the 1850s would prove to be the beginning of the boom, for cats would be seen everywhere until the late 1920s." Pictures of cats were seen on advertisements for "soap, thread boxes, games, hosiery, stove cleaners, rat poison, oils, and cigar boxes." Indeed, cigars became strongly associated with cats with the introduction of the "Me-ow Label in 1886, Tabby Cigars in 1894, Old Tom in 1900, White Cat in 1908, and Pussy in 1910–1916" [28].

5.3   The Cats of Writers and Artists

The respectability of cats was also accelerated during the late nineteenth and early twentieth centuries by their continued embrace by writers and artists. In England an important contributor was Beatrice Potter who in 1902 had published *The Tale of Peter Rabbit* which became a classic. In 1907 she followed this with *The Tale of Tom Kitten*, a study about a mother cat—Tabitha Twitchit—and her three children, Tom and his sisters Moppet and Mittens. Subsequently Potter published a *Tom Kitten* painting book for children, and Tom and other characters in the story were merchandised as toys. *The Tale of Tom Kitten* reinforced the emerging belief that cats were especially appropriate companions for small children. As the French writer Champfleury noted, "The cat is the nurse's favorite animal, and the first living creature where utterances strikes the ear of infancy...a baby falls asleep with a fantastic image of the cat impressed upon its brain" [29].

Just as the writers extolled the virtues of cats in the nineteenth and early twentieth centuries, so too did the artists. Champfleury had written: "Refined and delicate natures understand the cat. Women, poets and artists hold it in great esteem, for they recognize the exquisite delicacy of its nervous system." Similarly, Caroline Bugler noted: "It has always been the cat's personality, behavior and sensuality that has fascinated the most advanced painters, literary figures and musicians" [30, 31].

Among the best-known paintings of this period that included cats were those of Pierre-Auguste Renoir. His "Woman with a Cat" (1874), "Sleeping Girl with a Cat" (1880) (Fig. 5.2), and "Julie Manet with a Cat" (1887) are examples. Other French

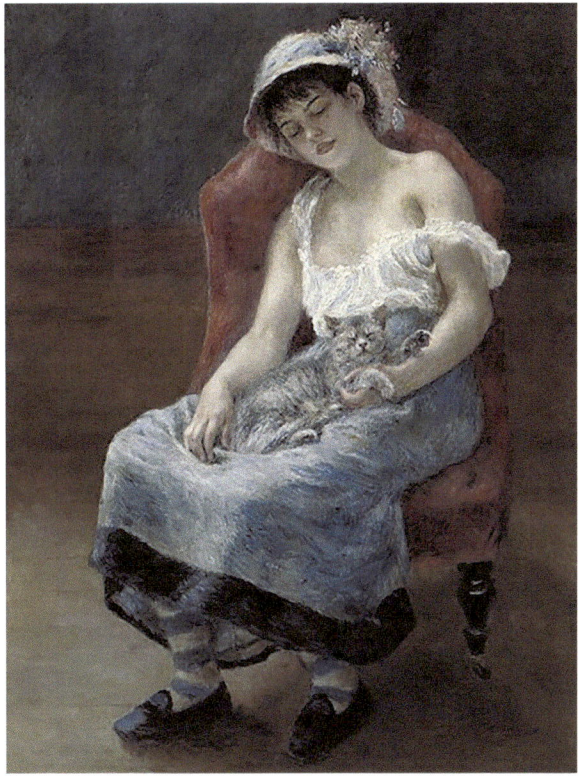

Fig. 5.2 Pierre-Auguste Renoir, "Sleeping Girl", 1880, Oil on canvas. Renoir included cats in other female portraits as well. (Image courtesy of The Clark Art Institute, Williamstown, MA, 1955.598, www.clarkart. edu Public Domain.)

Impressionists such as Berthe Moriset's "Young Girl with a Cat," (1892) and Pierre Bonard's "Woman with a Cat," (1912) also juxtaposed young women and cats. Philip Steer, among the few English Impressionists, also painted an elegant woman with her cat in "Hydrangeas" (1901).

5.4   Increasing Insanity

Claims that madness was increasing in England had been widespread even before King George III had become insane in 1788, and his illness exacerbated such fears. In 1792 clergyman and physician William Pargeter, in response to the king's illness, published his *Observations on Maniacal Disorders*. He described insanity as "the hideous malady which so amazingly prevails at this day" and said that "the frequency of this disease renders it truly alarming. . . . [it] has arrived at the height of its dominion." His eloquent description of the consequences of insanity is worth quoting:

> It would be almost too shocking to portray the real features of this terrible complaint . . . the situation of a fellow creature destitute of the guidance of that governing principle, reason—which chiefly distinguishes us from the inferior animals around us. . . . View man deprived

of that noble endowment, and see in how melancholy a posture he appears. He retains indeed the outward figure of the human species, but like the ruins of a once magnificent edifice, it only serves to remind us of his former dignity, and fills us with gloomy reflections of the loss of it [32].

Among the best-known English physicians in the closing years of the eighteenth century was Bethlem Hospital's John Haslam, labeled by British psychiatrist Denis Leigh as "by far the most original and discerning writer on psychiatry in the period 1798 to 1828." In 1798 Haslam published his *Observations on Insanity*, which was widely circulated throughout Europe and issued in a second edition in 1809, at which time it was also praised in the popular *Quarterly Review*. Haslam noted that "the alarming increase of insanity, as might naturally be expected, has incited many persons to an investigation of this disease. . . . In our own country more books on insanity have been published than in any other" [33–35].

Haslam was especially impressed by the increasing number of individuals who were becoming insane at a young age. In 1789 Andrew Harper, in *The Economy of Health: A Treatise on the Real Cause and Cure of Insanity*, had written "that young people are hardly ever liable to insanity and that the attack of this malady seldom happens before an advanced period of life." Yet Haslam described cases of this form of insanity as if they were something comparatively new: "There is a form of insanity which occurs in young persons. . . . This disorder commences about, or shortly after, the period of menstruation." Haslam proceeded to provide the first unequivocal English description of what we now label schizophrenia and in 1810 published an entire book on another case, *Illustrations of Madness: Exhibiting a Singular Case of Insanity* [36, 37].

In addition to describing schizophrenia, Haslam also provided remarkably clear descriptions of bipolar disorder (including the rapid-cycling kind), postpartum psychosis, postvaccinal encephalitis presenting with psychosis, alcoholic psychosis, and psychosis secondary to syphilis. Haslam's *Observations on Insanity* was judged by Denis Leigh to be "a most outstanding piece of work, surpassing in merit any previous publication both in England or on the continent" [38].

In the opening years of the nineteenth century, the consensus of Pargeter and Haslam was echoed by many of their colleagues. In his *Practical Observations on Insanity*, Joseph Cox noted that "insanity is unfortunately not only frequent but said to be peculiarly endemical to England." William Stark added that the loss of reason is "the heaviest calamity incident to our race." Thomas Trotter claimed that "the last century has been remarkable for the increase of a class of disease but little known in former times" and estimated that "nervous disorders" had replaced fevers as the most common affliction. And in 1808 John Reid, a London physician, wrote in the *Monthly* magazine that "the English malady, by its visible and rapid progression, renders itself every day more deserving of the title…Madness strides like a Colossus over the island" [39–42].

By this time parliament had also become concerned and, for the first time in English history, appointed the "Select Committee of the House of Commons, appointed to inquire into the state of lunatics." The impetus for parliament's actions was claims that insanity was increasing as well as an increasing number of highly publicized acts by mad people. The most egregious of these was James Hadfield's attempted killing of King George III in 1800. At his trial Hadfield said that he had done so by God's command to bring about the Second Coming; the irony of a mad-man attacking the king who was himself intermittently mad was not lost on the public. Hadfield was confined to Bethlem Hospital where he demonstrated his con-tinuing dangerousness by killing another patient.

The parliamentary hearings of the Select Committee in 1807 focused on the number of insane people in England, especially those being held in workhouses and jails. The sheriff of Gloucestershire, for example, testified that he had seen "poor lunatics who have been fastened to the leg of a table within a dwelling house; others chained to a post in an outhouse." He noted an increasing number of insane persons being held in jails and added: "I think jails, however well regulated, are places highly improper for the custody, and inconsistent with the cure of lunatics" [43].

The Select Committee in 1807 also attempted to collect data from each county regarding the total number of mad people in workhouses and jails. The results, how-ever, were highly variable and unreliable. It was clear that many counties were unwilling to share information with parliament on what had been regarded up to that time as a local problem. Some counties claimed that they had no insane persons at all in workhouses or jails, and others listed only a fraction of them. For example, Norfolk claimed to have 22 such people but an independent second count found 112. In 1810 Richard Powell, secretary of the commissioners of the College of Physicians, made another attempt to quantify the increasing insanity by using admissions to madhouses over time. In what was apparently the first statistical study of insanity, Powell showed a sharp rise in admissions between 1770 and 1809 and concluded that "the increase must actually have been very considerable, though we cannot ascertain its exact proportion" [44, 45].

The outcome of the Select Committee report was passage of "An Act for the Better Care and Maintenance of Lunatics," better known as the County Asylum Act of 1808, by which counties were encouraged, but not required, to build public insane asylums, to be paid for with local taxes. According to Leonard Smith, "the Act was remarkable in a number of ways, not least because it signified, whether by design or by accident, an unusually direct intervention by the state in health and welfare pro-vision." This was, it should be noted, the first of 20 parliamentary acts and amend-ments concerning insane persons, idiots, and insane asylums that would be passed during the nineteenth century. As John L. Crammer observed, "an astonishing amount of Parliamentary time was spent on this subject in the nineteenth century." Similarly, Vieda Skultans noted that "the number of Bills, reports of select commit-tees and inquiries relating to lunacy rose from a mere handful in the eighteenth century to seventy-one between the years 1801 and 1844" [46–48].

The first of the new county asylums opened in Nottinghamshire in 1812, fol-lowed by others in Bedfordshire, Norfolk, and Lancashire. By 1824 the number of county asylums had increased only to 8, ranging in size from 40 beds in Bedfordshire to 250 beds in Lancashire. The total number of beds in these county asylums was 932 to serve an 8-county total population of 3.4 million, suggesting that authorities expected utilization of the asylums to be low. And in some counties, it initially was; the Gloucestershire Asylum, which opened in 1823 with 110 beds, still had only 31 patients 6 months later [49].

In many counties, there was considerable resistance to building an asylum, both because of costs and because of doubts regarding need. The Gloucestershire Asylum, for example, had been first proposed in the 1790s but, because of local resistance, did not become a reality until 1823. In Middlesex, "several parishes lodged objections on grounds of cost," and those in the vicinity of the proposed asylum objected that the "cries and noises of the unhappy inmates" would be unsettling to them. In Suffolk there were "concerted local campaigns of petitions and protests" that delayed the asylum's opening [50].

In addition to the building of public asylums, private asylums also increased in the early years of the nineteenth century. In 1798 there had been 42 provincial and metropolitan "licensed houses," but by 1815 this number had increased to 72. Most of them were very small, and the annual admissions for all of them together averaged less than 500 a year until 1810–1815, when these admissions doubled.

5.5   What Was Causing the Increase?

Following the report of the Select Committee of 1807 and subsequent passage of the County Asylums Act, claims continued to be made that madness was increasing. Bryan Crowther, in *Practical Remarks*, published in 1811, called insanity "an affection so rapidly becoming prevalent among all orders of society." George Hill, in *An Essay on the Prevention and Cure of Insanity*, published in 1814, said that insanity "is certainly not to be rated among our declining diseases" and noted the contemporary outpouring of publications on the subject. Louis Simond, an American who made a 2-year tour of England in 1810 and 1811, published his observations in 1815, noting that "madness appears to be fatally common in Great Britain" and that this high incidence existed despite the fact that "the qualifications required for acknowledged insanity, are by no means easily attained in England, where a greater latitude is granted for whims, fancies, and eccentricities, than in other countries" [51–53].

Increasingly, however, in the early years of the nineteenth century, public discussion shifted from the question of whether madness was increasing to why it was increasing. A definitive answer to that question had been offered in 1782 by Thomas Arnold, an Edinburgh-trained physician who ran a private asylum in Leicester. His two-volume *Observations on the Nature, Kinds, Causes and Prevention of Insanity, Lunacy or Madness* was widely praised, including by James Boswell, and included a chapter on the question of increasing insanity.

Arnold acknowledged that "instances of Insanity are, at this day, amazingly numerous in this kingdom—probably more so than they ever were in any former period." The "most powerful causes" of insanity, Arnold claimed, were "religion, love, commerce, and the various passions which attend the desire, pursuit, and acquisition of riches—every species of luxury—and all violent and permanent attachments whatsoever." As evidence for his theory, Arnold compared England's high rate of insanity to that in France which had not yet had its revolution and which Arnold claimed had a much lower rate of insanity. According to Arnold, under French Catholicism, "whose chief characteristic is superstition," the "pardon for sins of all sorts and sizes is so easily obtained [as] in every popish country that few true believers . . . can be supposed to be much troubled with religious melancholy." Similarly, "love, with them, is almost wholly an affair of art;—it has more of fancy than passion; and is rather an amusement of the imagination, than a serious business of the heart." Regarding "the desire, and prospect, of acquiring riches . . . there can be but little hope of attaining riches in a land of slaves, where the bulk and strength of a nation is depressed and impoverished . . . being subject to the will of an absolute monarch," in contrast to England's "happy land of liberty." Arnold thus concluded: "All these circumstances being taken into the account, it seems not improbable that this disorder is not only much more prevalent in England than in France, but more peculiar to this than to any other country. For even waving the other considerations just enumerated, an excess of wealth and luxury, in which perhaps no nation upon earth can vie with this, seems to entitle us to an abundant share of the curse which appears too plainly to be entailed upon their possessors" [54].

It is surely a peculiar form of patriotism to view insanity as evidence of a superior civilization but that is what Arnold was arguing. Not only was insanity increasing, but the English should be proud of that fact. Arnold noted that "we hear of few or no instance of Insanity among barbarous nations, whether ancient or modern." Insanity was also rare, he claimed, in Scotland and in the poorer areas of Wales, regions in which "wealth and luxury are but little known." Insanity, in brief, was a marker of an advanced civilization [55].

Arnold's explanation for the increasing insanity became widely accepted in the closing years of the eighteenth and early nineteenth centuries. England's industrial revolution was expanding rapidly with a doubling of the real national output between 1780 and 1800 and a tenfold rise in patents for new inventions. Thus in 1788 William Rowley claimed that "in those kingdoms where the greatest luxuries, refinements, wealth, and unrestrained liberty abound, are the most numerous instances of madness." The following year Benjamin Falkner echoed both Arnold and Rowley: "The rapidity with which the disorder has spread over this country, within the last fifty years, may be attributed, in great measure, to the increase of luxury...Inordinate desires, and the indulgence of inordinate passions." In 1802 Thomas Beddeos spoke about nations "civilized enough to be capable of insanity." In 1816 David Uwins wrote that "luxury invites excess and excess spells madness...In proportion as man emerges from his primeval state, do the Furies of disease advance upon him." In 1824 Alexander Morison noted that "insanity increases with civilization." Finally, in 1837, William A.F. Browne agreed that "with luxury, indeed, insanity appears to keep equal pace" [56–60].

5.6   Madness Among "the Better Sort"

As the discussion of increasing madness became widespread in nineteenth-century England, there was agreement that some groups of people were more affected than others. This had been noted as early as 1733 when George Cheyne in *The English Malady* singled out people "of the better sort" as being most susceptible to insanity, specifically "those of the liveliest and quickest natural Parts, whose Faculties are the brightest and most spiritual, and whose Genius is most keen and penetrating, and particularly where there is the most delicate Sensation and Taste, both of Pleasure and Pain." Others at that time had similarly claimed that "lords and ladies, accustomed to luxurious living and idleness…were more liable to what we call neuroses and psychoses than people in the lower ranks" [61].

Echos of Cheyne continued to be heard in the nineteenth century. Lord Simond, the American who visited England, was told that "the rich particularly are most exposed to this calamity [insanity]…madness appears to be fatally common…among the higher ranks." English psychiatrist W.A.F. Browne claimed that the rural poor "is to a great degree exempt from insanity" but the wealthy and educated are especially susceptible because they are exposed to "excitement…and to the formation of habits of thought and action inimical to the preservation of serenity and health." Similarly David Uwins in his book on mental disorders singled out the intellectual avant-garde as being most affected—those who had "pianos, parasols, Edinburgh Reviews, and Paris-going desires." The French were making similar claims. Esquirol claimed that madness was more usually a disease of the rich, while Phillipe Pinel noted that the large asylum in Paris contained a disproportionate number of "priests and monks" as well as "many artists, painters, sculptors and musicians [and] some poets extasized by their own productions" [62–65].

An interest in, and/or personal experience with, madness was endemic among English writers and poets in the nineteenth century. Such interest was presaged in 1796 when Mary Lamb, in an acute attack of mania, killed her mother with a carving knife as they were preparing dinner. Mary, age 31, had had one previous manic episode and suffered additional attacks every year or two for the remainder of her life. Between hospitalizations Mary was cared for at home by her younger brother, Charles, who himself had been hospitalized for a manic attack at age 19 and thereafter had problems with alcohol abuse. Charles and Mary were both writers, he as a widely read essayist whose whimsical creations included "A Dissertation upon Roast Pig" and "A Chapter on Ears." Together they wrote *Tales Founded on the Plays of Shakespeare* for children, and Mary published a book on *Poetry for Children*. The specter of madness was ever present for them both. At one point Charles Lamb wrote to his closest friend, Samuel Taylor Coleridge: "Dream not, Coleridge, of having tasted all of the grandeur and wildness of Fancy, till you have gone mad. All now seems to me vapid; comparatively so" [66–68].

Coleridge also had a deep interest in madness, experiencing periods of depression and having been discharged from the army as being insane. The correspondence between Lamb and Coleridge often touched on madness and the mental state of their colleagues; for example, "Coleridge, you will rejoice to hear that Cowper is recovered from his lunacy" (May 1776). Coleridge's two best known poems, "Kubla Khan" and "The Rime of the Ancient Mariner," are both said to be about madness. As early as 1813, George Crabbe said of "The Ancient Mariner": "It does not describe Madness by its Effects but by Imitation, as if a painter to give a picture of Lunacy should make his Canvas crazy, and fill it with wild unconnected Limbs and Distortions of features . . ." And Michael Shimer wrote: "The Mariner as a mad figure need hardly be argued. So strange is his appearance, behavior, and power that little or no doubt is left to his marked abnormality. . . . The theme of madness originates, of course, in the Mariner's killing of the albatross. . . . It is a manifestation of human irrationality." In his correspondence, Coleridge likened madness to "a fiery hell":

> Why need we talk of a fiery hell? If the will, which is the law of our nature, were withdrawn from our memory, fancy, understanding, and reason, no other hell could equal, for a spiritual being, what we should then feel, from the anarchy of our powers. It would be conscious madness—a horrid thought!

For much of his life, Coleridge was also addicted to opium [69–72].

William Wordsworth, England's poet laureate from 1843 to 1850, was close friends with both Lamb and Coleridge, and it was he who suggested to Coleridge to have the Ancient Mariner kill the albatross. Wordsworth was himself subject to periods of depression and was drawn to the subject of insanity. According to Michael Shimer, "During the mental crisis in his own life (roughly between the spring of 1795 and the fall of 1797), Wordsworth wrote a group of poems that explicitly deal with the theme of madness." One of them was titled "The Mad Mother":

> A fire was once within my brain;
> And in my head a dull, dull, pain;
> And fiendish faces one, two, three,
> Hung at my breasts, and pulled at me [73].

Robert Southey, poet laureate for 30 years, was Coleridge's brother-in-law. At his home in the Lake Country, he entertained many of the poets of his generation. Among Southey's most popular poems was "Mary, The Maid of the Inn" about a woman who becomes mad. Originally titled "Mary the Maniac," it was widely reprinted in contemporary magazines. Ironically, Southey's wife became insane and spent 3 years in an asylum.

Madness was a major theme in the life of William Blake. Charles Lamb referred to him as "the mad Wordsworth." Southey, after meeting Blake, said: "You could not have delighted in him—his madness was too evident." Whether or not Blake was truly insane has been debated endlessly by his biographers; what is clear is that he regularly experienced visions and communed with spirits. Paul Youngquist argued that Blake "was a poet for whom madness became a major subject. . . . Blake made poetry out of pathology. . . . Madness emerges in his poetry as a thematic preoccupation." *The Four Zoas*, which was not published in Blake's lifetime, has been described as "a mythological investigation of madness" with "contemporary clinical parallels in the symptomology of schizophrenia" [74].

Blake was also very interested in the eighteenth-century poets Thomas Chatterton, who committed suicide, and William Cowper, who became insane. He collaborated with Cowper's biographer to produce illustrations for the book. Blake also painted a clearly mad Nebuchadnezzar, based on the biblical Book of Daniel. For "Jerusalem," Blake's greatest poem, one biographer suggested that he incorporated "the shade of Cowper" into the specter that torments the protagonist [75].

George Crabbe, originally trained as a surgeon, became a successful poet and friend of Wordsworth, Byron, and Scott. In 1796 Crabbe's wife became insane following the birth of their third child, and thereafter insanity became a major theme in his work. Among his many portrayals of insanity was "Sir Eustace Grey"; published in 1807, it was set in a madhouse and included extended descriptions of a madman's hallucinations. The poem was "well received in its day," and a reviewer noted: "Mr. Crabbe has, perhaps, been driven to the melancholy contemplation on insanity in all its wild variety of mood, and so, alas! to our misfortune, have we." "Tales," published in 1812, was another portrait of insanity [76–78].

Like Crabbe, John Keats initially trained in medicine before giving it up to be a poet. In *Touched with Fire*, Kay Jamison described Keats' mood swings and speculated that he might have had bipolar disorder before he died from tuberculosis at 25. According to Shiner, Keats' literary ballad "La Belle Dame Sans Merci" concerns a "noble mind that has gone mad." Keats also wrote an "Ode on Melancholy" [79].

George Gordon, Lord Byron, was one of the most influential of the English Romantic poets. His close friend Sir Walter Scott wrote of him: "There is something dreadful in reflecting that one gifted so much above his fellow-creatures should thus labour under some strange mental malady that destroys his peace of mind and happiness. . . ." Byron's "strange mental malady" was bipolar disorder; throughout his life he suffered from periods of recurrent mania and severe depression, and he ultimately was divorced by his wife on the grounds that he was insane. During one period of depression, he contemplated suicide but was stopped by the realization that "it would have given pleasure to my mother-in-law." The fear of impending insanity haunted Byron, as he wrote to a friend: "I don't know that I shan't end with insanity, for I find a want of method in arranging my thoughts that perplexes me strangely." This preoccupation with madness was reflected in his poetry, as in his description of an insane woman in *The Dream*. Reflecting on his own madness and that of his fellow poets, Byron said: "We of the craft are all crazy" [80].

In 1816, Byron met Percy Bysshe Shelley. Shelley found Byron "exceedingly interesting" but "mad as the winds." Shelley, in fact, had his own psychiatric problems, including recurrent episodes of depression and apparent hallucinations. Kay Jamison, in *Touched with Fire*, argued that Shelley, like Byron, had bipolar disorder, although some Shelley scholars do not agree. Shelley and Byron spent much time together between 1816 and 1821, during which time Shelley wrote *Julian and Maddalo*, a poem about two men (thought to be Shelley and Byron themselves) who visit a friend who has become insane and is incarcerated in a madhouse:

...The clap of tortured hands,
Fierce yells and howlings and lamentings keen,
And laughter where complaint had merrier been,
Moans, shrieks, and curses, and blaspheming prayers,
Accosted us [81].

Sir Walter Scott was friends with many of the Romantic poets and one of the most widely read writers of his era. Although he suffered from the "black dog" of melancholy, Scott was never insane. However, he "made mental maladies a special study" and immortalized insane women, most prominently as Madge Wildfire in *The Heart of Midlothian* (1818) and as Lucy Ashton in *The Bride of Lammermoor* (1819). In the former, Madge is referred to as "Madge of Bedlam" and sings of her time spent there:

In the bonny cells of Bedlam
Ere I was ane and twenty,
I had hempen bracelets strong,
And merry whips, ding-dong,
And prayer and fasting plenty.

One scholar labeled this scene "one of the most poignant scenes in all of Scott's fiction, here is insanity on display . . . the face of madness grimacing at the sane world." Another of Sir Walter Scott's mad heroines, Lucy Ashton, was subsequently the heroine of eight different operas, most notably Gaetano Donizetti's *Lucia di Lammermoor* (1835), in which Lucia suffers from visual and auditory hallucinations. In the "mad scene," Lucia, overtly insane, kills the man she has just been forced to marry [82–84].

John Clare was a promising young poet specializing in poems of rural England when he developed psychosis. In 1837 he was voluntarily admitted to Dr. Matthew Allen's private asylum in Essex. He experienced auditory hallucinations and grandiose delusions in which he believed himself to be Lord Byron, Lord Nelson, or other famous persons. He told one visitor, "They have cut off my head and picked out all the letters of the alphabet—all the vowels and consonants—and brought them out through my ears." Clare spent 4 years at Dr. Allen's asylum and then 23 additional years at the Northamptonshire Lunatic Asylum, which he characterized as "the land of Sodom where all the people's brains are turned the wrong way." During his extended stay in these asylums, Clare continued writing poems, some of which reflected his despair at being confined and forgotten [85–87].

During the 4 years when John Clare lived at Dr. Allen's private asylum in Essex, Alfred Lord Tennyson lived a short walk away. At the time Tennyson was regarded as one of England's most promising young poets; he would later be appointed poet laureate from 1850 to 1892. Tennyson had purposefully moved to be near Dr. Allen's asylum to get psychiatric care for one brother, Septimus. Another brother, Edgar, had already become insane and would be hospitalized for 57 years in the York Asylum. According to one biographer "from the time Tennyson was a child...the specter of madness was always to hover over him and often to come dangerously near." He regularly visited Dr. Allen's asylum to "study the ravings of the demented at firsthand" and almost certainly would have had conversations with his fellow poet, John Clare. Later Tennyson used mad figures in several of his poems, including "Maud" which was his "favorite poem and one which he loved to recite." A contemporary reviewer described "Maud" as "neither more nor less than the autobiography of a madman...depicted by the hand of a master." And Michael Shimer, in his study of madness in nineteenth-century English poetry, claimed that "the madhouse section of 'Maud'...is probably the most realistic portrayal of insanity that we shall encounter in our study" [88, 89].

Madness is also prominent in Charlotte Bronte's 1847 novel *Jane Eyre*. The heroine goes to Thornfield Hall as a governess and falls in love with the master of the house, Edward Rochester. He proposes marriage, but Jane discovers that he is already wed to an insane woman who is being hidden in the attic. Bronte's description of Mrs. Rochester is that of a dangerous wild animal: "In the deep shade, at the farther end of the room, a figure ran backwards and forwards. What it was, whether beast or human being, one could not, at first sight, tell: it grovelled, seemingly, on all fours; it snatched and growled like some strange wild animal: but it was covered with clothing, and a quantity of dark, grizzled hair, wild as a mane, hid its head and face" [90].

When Charlotte Bronte was later criticized for her brutish depiction of Mrs. Rochester, she responded that she was merely reflecting the reality of some cases of madness "in which all that is good or even human seems to disappear from the mind and a fiend-like nature replaces it." Such a description was consistent with the increasing tenor of the times. As Ann Colley noted in *Tennyson and Madness*, "Brontë's Mrs. Rochester, locked within the tower of Thornfield Hall," was not merely "a literary convention" but rather reflected that period's preoccupation with madness, "a madness that was a pressing and threatening reality" [91, 92].

An ironic postscript to *Jane Eyre* was Charlotte Bronte's dedication of the second edition of the book to William Makepeace Thackeray, whom she greatly admired. Unknown to Bronte, Thackeray's wife, Isabella, who had become insane, tried to drown their daughter, and attempted suicide, was being quietly confined in a house in London under the care of two women attendants. Both Mrs. Rochester and Mrs. Thackeray became mad 4 years following their marriages, "both were given to manic bursts of laughter" and "both were at times violent and even homicidal." When Charlotte Bronte learned of Isabella Thackeray's condition, she "was torn between amazement and mortification," apologized to Thackeray, and told a friend that it proved that "fact is often stranger than fiction" [93].

Among all the nineteenth-century poets and writers with an interest in madness, however, none surpassed Charles Dickens. He visited asylums regularly, including asylums in New York and Boston during his 1842 visit to America. He was also remarkably knowledgeable about insanity. His personal library included Robert Burton's *Anatomy of Melancholy*, John Conolly's *On Some Forms of Insanity*, Forbes Winslow's *The Incubation of Insanity*, and W. C. Hood's *Suggestions for the Future Provision of Criminal Lunatics* [85–87]. The two journals Dickens edited, *Household Words* and *All the Year Round*, regularly included articles on madhouses and asylum reform. Most importantly, Dickens was close friends with John Conolly, one of the foremost psychiatrists of the mid-nineteenth century, and with two of the lunacy commissioners, Bryan Proctor and John Forster, whose full-time jobs were to inspect madhouses. Forster, in fact, became Dickens's first biographer with his *Life of Charles Dickens* in 1872. It is likely that the ideas for many of Dickens's mad characters were derived from his conversations with these men [94].

The most notable mad character created by Dickens was published in 1837 as "A Madman's Manuscript," one of the monthly installments of *The Pickwick Papers.* The story is a strange tale, told in the first person by a madhouse inmate who is being laughed at by visitors peering into his cell. Rather than feeling humiliated, the madman delights in his status and in his ability to terrify others: "Show me the monarch whose angry frown was ever feared like the glare of a madman's eye. . . . Ho! Ho! It's a grand thing to be mad!" He then recounts the onset of his illness, "watching the progress of the fever that was to consume [his] brain," the voices screaming in his ears, his attempted murder of his young wife, and then his success-ful murder of his brother-in-law and subsequent incarceration [95].

In *Barnaby Rudge*, published 4 years later, Dickens continued this theme. According to one critic, "madness is loosed upon the text from the onset. . . . The novel is, in that sense, a meditation on the perils of growing insanity, insanity always threatening to erupt in violence, and the impotence of traditional asylums such as Bethlem Hospital to cope with that growth." In the novel a rumor is spread that a mob, led by Lord Byron, who himself is depicted in the book as having the symp-toms of insanity, "meant to throw the gates of Bedlam open, and let all the madmen loose. This suggested such dreadful images to people's minds, and was indeed an act so fraught with new and unimaginable horrors in the contemplation, that it beset them more than any loss or cruelty of which they could foresee the worst, and drove many sane men nearly mad themselves" [96, 97].

Charles Dickens continued to depict mad characters in his novels throughout his career. One of the best known is *David Copperfield's* Mr. Dick, who believes he has things in his head that came from the head of King Charles I and were transferred to him when the king was beheaded in 1649. In 1851 Dickens visited St. Luke's Asylum in London shortly after Christmas, later publishing a description of the holiday dance held for patients as "A Curious Dance Round a Curious Tree," in which he praised the nonuse of restraints as part of the increasingly popular moral treatment. And in 1857, in *The Lazy Tour of Two Idle Apprentices*, published with Willkie Collins, Dickens described a fictional visit to an insane asylum, including a poignant description of patients standing idly on the wards of the asylum: "Long groves of blighted men-and-women trees; interminable avenues of hopeless faces; numbers, without the slightest power of really combining for any earthly purpose; a society of human creatures who have nothing in common but that they have all lost the power of being humanly social with one another" [98, 99].

Willkie Collins, with whom Dickens wrote *The Lazy Tour of Two Idle Apprentices* was well known in his time as the author of what were called sensation novels. According to David Oberhelman's thesis on the Victorian novel, these novels exhib-ited "a mania for madness itself, . . . producing a veritable Bedlam of madmen and madwomen. . . . Madness and the system of private lunatic asylums . . . are almost ubiquitous plot elements in the sensation novels. . . . Wrongful confinement . . . , the corruption of 'mad-doctors,' and the threat of hereditary madness become some of the most lurid nightmares [in the works of Willkie Collins and his contemporaries]" [100].

Collins' best-known novel was *The Woman in White* about a woman who escapes from an asylum. It was so popular that it created new marketing strategies, including a line of *Women in White* clothing and perfume. *Armadale*, published by Collins in 1866, is about "Dr. Downward," an unethical psychiatrist who confines people inappropriately in his private asylum. According to Oberhelman "various aspects of madness dominate the prose of the text. . . . Madness so saturates the text that any debate over figurative or literal uses of the term is rendered meaningless. . . . It illustrates the true epidemic proportions of madness in the 1800s" [101].

Another widely read sensation novel of the early 1860s was *Lady Audley's Secret*, written by Mary Elizabeth Braddon. Mrs. Braddon had a special interest in insanity, since she was living with, but could not marry, publisher John Maxwell, whose wife was insane and confined to an asylum. In Mrs. Braddon's book, the "secret" is that Lady Audley is insane, a fact slowly revealed in the novel through her bigamy and subsequent murder of one of her husbands. In her confession at the end of the book, Lady Audley says: "I killed him because I AM MAD! because my intellect is a little way on the wrong side of that narrow boundary-line between sanity and insanity" [102, 103].

Although most of the available evidence regarding madness among "the better sort" comes from writers, especially poets and novelists, there were also a few artists who became mad in the late eighteenth and early nineteenth centuries. John Robert Cozens was a well-known British watercolorist who became psychotic at age 42, was hospitalized in Bethlem Hospital, and died 3 years later. Lemuel Abbott, a prominent portrait painter whose painting of Lord Nelson hangs at 10 Downing Street, was declared insane at age 38 and treated by Dr. Thomas Munro. James Gillray, a caricaturist who had been called "the father of the political cartoon," became suicidal and psychotic at age 57 although alcohol abuse was a contributing factor. Finally, Richard Dadd, regarded as one of Britain's most promising young artists, developed a paranoid psychosis at age 25 and in 1842 killed his father, who he believed to be the devil in disguise. He continued painting, including a work that hangs at the Tate Gallery, while hospitalized until his death at age 68 [104].

5.7   Was Insanity Really Increasing?

During the middle years of the nineteenth century, as English writers were incorporating madness into their writings and, in some cases, experiencing it, the question of whether or not insanity was increasing came again to the fore. The immediate precipitant was a claim in 1820 that, contrary to popular beliefs, madness was *not* increasing. The person who made the claim was George Man Burrows, a prominent London physician who ran a private madhouse in Chelsea. Burrows was deeply involved in establishing the legal rights of the medical profession and had played a leading role in persuading parliament to pass the Apothecaries Act of 1815 which gave physicians control over the prescribing of medicines. Burrows also fought to establish insanity as the legal province of physicians. Thus he had both a professional and a financial interest in demonstrating the success of the medical profession in caring for the mad. Increasing insanity clearly would not be good for the reputation of the profession [105, 106].

In his 1820 book entitled *An Inquiry Into Certain Errors Relative to Insanity* and in *Commentaries*, published 8 years later, Burrows reviewed available data on the number of insane persons in England and Ireland and concluded that the total number was approximately 6,000, similar to the estimate derived for England from the Select Committee survey of 1807. He acknowledged that "foreigners of all countries pronounce insanity as the opprobrium of England" and that "the popular opinion is that insanity is alarmingly prevalent." He argued strongly, however, that insanity was "not an increasing malady" and in 1828 even argued that it was decreasing in incidence [107].

Burrows offered two reasons for his belief that insanity was not increasing. The first was the fact that insane asylums, presumably including the one he owned, were effective in treating this condition, and therefore, ipso facto, insanity had to be decreasing. He explained it as follows: "I have, therefore, no other ground for my conviction of the general diminution in the number of lunatics, than the pleasing and incontrovertible fact, that wherever asylums for insane persons have been established, from the superior mode of treatment, both medical and moral, the number who recover is much greater than heretofore; and, consequently, that the aggregate number of the insane must be lessened." Burrows's second reason for denying any increase in insanity—and even arguing for a decrease—was that increasing insanity would be a national scandal and therefore it *should* not be true: "Hence, as the respective exciting causes vary, so likewise must everywhere the number of lunatics. But does it thence follow that insanity must be increasing? A conclusion so humiliating cannot be entertained without the most painful reflections; nor, if it be really so, can the consequences be indifferent, even in a national point of view?" [108]

Burrows's conclusions were quoted by some contemporary psychiatrists and others who did not believe, or did not want to believe, that insanity was increasing. More than 150 years later, historians Ida Macalpine and Richard Hunter, in *George III and the Mad Business*, would cite Burrows as having definitively proven that insanity had not increased in the early nineteenth century: "The question whether insanity was on the increase Dr. Burrows therefore answered with a definite no. . . . This particular ghost had at last been laid to rest and was not heard from again." This declaration was a surprising error for Macalpine and Hunter, whose scholarship is generally beyond reproach; in fact, in the 1820s, the ghost of increasing insanity was just beginning to walk the land [108, 109].

In contrast to the support he received, Burrows was also widely criticized by contemporary reviewers who did not agree with him. An anonymous reviewer in the 1821 *Quarterly Review*, for example, criticized Burrows's equating of suicide with insanity: "We question too the propriety of making the number of suicides an indication of the number of the insane, since we are not disciples of that creed which indiscriminately puts down every case of self-destruction to the score of deranged intellect." Burrows's second book on insanity was subjected to a scathing review in the same journal, where it was dismissed as "a mass of trash" and "a wretched compilation of scraps, gathered from all sorts of sources, and full of inaccuracies. . . . The author, in truth, undertook a task to which his mind was totally unequal. . . ." [110, 111]

Burrow's claim that insanity was not increasing in England continued to be a minority view for the following four decades. A major reason for this was the publication by Sir Andrew Halliday of a *Report of the Number of Lunatics and Idiots in England and Wales* in 1829, 1 year after the publication of Burrow's second book. Halliday was an Edinburgh-trained physician who had participated in the 1807 census of the insane and then continued to collect data for the next 20 years. He had served as a physician in the Royal Navy, including being at the Battle of Waterloo when the Napoleonic forces were defeated, and had been knighted in 1821. He had also become the personal physician to William, duke of Clarence and St. Andrews, who in 1830 became King William IV. Halliday was regarded as one of the most knowledgeable professionals concerning the census of the insane and, since he was not connected to a public or private asylum, also one of the most credible.

In his report Halliday divided the insane into "lunatics" (developed insanity after childhood) and "idiots" (insane since birth) and counted separately those in asylums, those in workhouses, and those being kept at home. His preliminary count was 6,806 lunatics and 5,741 idiots, or 12,547 total, but he acknowledged that this was an undercount and estimated the true total at 16,500. Assuming the same proportion of lunatics to idiots in the uncounted portion of the total, the total number of lunatics in Halliday's estimate would have been 8,941, or approximately 0.79 per 1,000 total population. This figure showed, Halliday concluded, that "insanity, in all its forms, prevails to a most alarming extent in England. . . . The numbers of the afflicted have become more than tripled during the last twenty years!" He added that it was no longer possible to dispute these "melancholy facts" and that it would be "a consciousness of criminal negligence were one to attempt longer to conceal them" [112].

Halliday also thought he knew why insanity was increasing. The cause, he said, was "over exertion of the mind, in overworking its instruments so as to weaken them . . . the derangement of the vital functions, that re-act upon the brain, and derange its operation." He contrasted the large number of lunatics in England with their paucity among "the savage tribes of men; not one of our African travellers remark having seen a single madman" [113].

Over the next two decades, other physicians supported Halliday's conclusion. In 1835, for example, James C. Prichard published his *Treatise on Insanity and Other Disorders Affecting the Mind* in which he carefully assessed the data on insanity collected by the 1807 census as well as the work of Burrows and Halliday. Prichard was a Bristol physician who was widely respected for his 1813 book, *Researches into the Physical History of Man*, in which he speculated on the origin of the races and was among the first to suggest that humans had originated in Africa. After examining all of the evidence regarding increasing insanity, Prichard concluded that "the apparent increase is everywhere so striking that it leaves on the mind a strong suspicion that cases of insanity are far more numerous than formerly" [114].

In 1837 another prominent physician strongly supported Halliday's conclusion that madness was on the increase. William A.F. Browne, a Scottish physician, was a friend of Charles Darwin and author of *What Asylums Were, Are and Ought to Be.* According to sociologist Andrew Scull, Browne's book was "enormously influential" and made Browne "among the four or five most prominent British alienists of his generation." Regarding insanity, Browne claimed "that a much greater number of cases is known to exist, and to require treatment, than formerly," and that the increase was far more rapid than the population in general. The reason for this increase, according to Browne, was that "as we recede, step by step, from the simple...manners of our ancestors, and advance in industry and knowledge and happiness, this malignant persecutor strides onward, signalizing every era...by an increase, a new hecatomb, of victims" [115].

In 1843 the first census of insane persons was carried out since Halliday's report in 1829. It found 14,792 "lunatics" in public and private asylums, workhouses, and private dwellings. Based on the total population of England, the rate of insanity was thus 0.93 per 1,000 people. In 1829 Halliday had reported a total of 8,941 insane persons, or 0.79 per 1,000 population. Thus during the 14 years, there had been an 18 percent increase in insanity, supporting the claims of Halliday, Prichard, Browne, and others.

One of the interesting findings from the 1843 census was that insanity in England was not evenly distributed. Nine counties in Southern England and the Midlands (Gloucestershire, Oxfordshire, Berkshire, Wiltshire, Hampshire, Dorset, Somerset, Devonshire, and Cornwall) had a rate of insane persons per 1,000 total population of 0.46 to 0.89, with an average of 0.65. Three of these counties (Wiltshire 0.89, Hampshire 0.84, and Dorset 0.76) were among the four English counties with the highest rates of insanity and are contiguous. The eight northernmost counties, by contrast, had a rate of insane persons per 1,000 total population of 0.29 to 0.52, with an average of 0.42. These included the four counties with the lowest rates (Lancashire 0.38, Cheshire 0.33, Staffordshire 0.39, and Derbyshire 0.29) and are also contiguous. Thus, insanity in England in 1843 appeared to be most prevalent in the south and the Midlands and to become less prevalent as one moved north. It was a pattern that would be seen repeatedly later in the century [116].

In addition to the 1843 census, there were other indications that insanity was increasing at this time. The number of private insane asylums had increased from 72 in 1815 to 149 in 1849, and the size of many of them had doubled or more. The first eight public asylums, opened by 1823, had an average of 116 beds, "but almost at once it became clear that the number of beds needed had been seriously underestimated in most areas, and the asylums grew rapidly in size." For example, the asylum at Lancashire was built in 1816 for 250 patients, but by 1844 it held 600. The Nottinghamshire Asylum increased from 80 to 206 beds, and the Bedfordshire Asylum nearly quadrupled in size from 40 to 139 beds between 1812 and 1844. Additional asylums were built, including the Middlesex Asylum at Hanwell, with

1,000 beds to serve London, but they were filled as soon as the doors were opened [117].

It should be noted that the increase in asylum population in the second quarter of the nineteenth century occurred despite high death rates in the asylums. At the Lancashire Asylum, cholera killed 94 patients in 1832, and influenza killed 46 more in 1837. At the Wakefield Asylum, influenza killed 30 in 1837, and cholera killed over 100 in 1849. The death rate for new admissions to the Hanwell Asylum was 18 percent in the first year, reflecting the fact that many admissions also had serious medical, as well as psychiatric, problems [118].

Still another measure of the increasing insanity was the number of forensic cases, called criminal lunatics, being held in asylums. In 1837 they totaled 138 for all of England but by 1847 they had increased to 337. Such numbers surprised nobody since people had been observing an increasing number of high-profile, violent acts by insane person. In 1812, for example, John Bellingham, paranoid and insane, had shot Prime Minister Spencer Percival in the lobby of the House of Commons. In 1829 an insane Jonathan Martin had set fire to the York Cathedral. In 1840 Edward Oxford shot at Queen Victoria's carriage and was subsequently declared insane. Three years later, Daniel M'Naghten shot Edward Drummond, mistaking him for Prime Minister Robert Peel. Indeed, according to one historian of this period, "it would be safe to say that a majority feared that madness was spreading in epidemic proportions from man to man, from generation to generation, and from region to region. Many saw madness as a monster lying beneath the surface, waiting to be given an opportunity to rise and consume their England" [119, 120].

As noted previously, there was considerable local resistance to the building of public asylums in England. In later years some historians, such as Michael Foucoult in *Madness and Civilization*, would argue that asylums were built as part of "the great confinement" of the insane, paupers, criminals, and vagrants who were not economically productive. The financing of asylums was, until 1874, the exclusive responsibility of local governments, which meant higher local taxes each time an asylum was built; after 1874 the central government contributed approximately 40 percent of the asylum costs.

Given such costs, it is not surprising that "ratepayer and taxpayer resistance to increased public expenditure was deep-rooted, vituperative, and often crippling." As early as 1859, the persistent calls by public officials to build new asylums and enlarge existing asylums were said to cause "terrible discouragement and complaint with the ratepayers." In Sussex "there was clearly a highly organized campaign against building a county asylum." In Buckinghamshire in 1849, "six hundred ratepayers, led by Benjamin Disraeli, renewed their opposition [to an asylum], complaining that they had already been taxed for a new jail and judges' lodging, and were now being asked to underwrite another expensive capital project." Disraeli was at the time a member of parliament for Buckinghamshire. An editorial in the *Westminster Review* complained of pianos and other "lavish expenditures" in public asylums: "It is no exaggeration to say that two-thirds of the permanent residents in every pauper asylum care little for the luxurious furnishings around them. A considerable proportion, indeed, could not tell the difference between a palace and a stable-yard" [121–127].

A large number of skirmishes in the battle over the costs of insanity took place regarding local workhouses. It was these institutions that had housed mentally ill individuals before the county asylums were built, and they did so at a cost of one half to one eighth the cost of asylum care. When county authorities were ordered to transfer mentally ill residents from the workhouses to the newly built asylums, they often transferred only the most disturbed and disturbing individuals and kept the rest in the workhouses. In 1828, for example, there were estimated to be approximately 9,000 "lunatics and idiots" in England's workhouses. This number decreased in the 1840s and early 1850s as more county asylums opened but then increased again by 1861 to almost 9,000, and by 1870 "workhouses held over 12,000 pauper lunatics, about 25 percent of their total number." By this time some county asylums, faced with marked overcrowding, were even quietly transferring some chronic and nonassaultive patients back to workhouses despite laws and official psychiatric rhetoric prohibiting such transfers [128–131].

In the 1850s, insanity increased faster than it had ever done. A national census carried out in 1854 reported a total of 30,538 insane persons, more than double the 14,792 reported in 1843. At the next census in 1859, the number had risen to 36,762. Even allowing for population growth insanity had doubled in 15 years from 0.93 per 1,000 population to 1.87 per 1000. Especially alarming was the suspicion that the insanity was disproportionately affecting "the better sort." According to Andrew Scull, "the best professional opinion suggested that it was the educated, the wealthy, the most cultural segments of the community…who had the most to fear from the spectre of madness" [132].

Many medical professionals continued to express concern. In 1848, in his book *Insanity Tested by Science*, Charles M. Burnett observed: "It has long been a popular opinion that insanity is a more common disease in our country than in any other, and that this opinion has of late years been strengthened by the assertion of many that the disease is on the increase." Two years later an author, identified only as "the late Medical Superintendent of an Asylum for the Insane," described insanity as "a great national evil, spreading through numerous families, in which every remedy that medical science can suggest, and law can enforce, ought immediately to be applied." In 1854 Alfred Maddox, the proprietor of an asylum in Kent, claimed that "in no other country, compared with England, do we find such numerous and formidable examples of this extensive scourge." And 3 years later, John Hawkes, a medical officer in the Wiltshire County Asylum, wrote that "the fair face of England, dotted over with her many public asylums for the relief and refuge of mental disease, presents a picture of rare and painful interest. . . . I doubt if ever the history of the world, or the experience of past ages, could show a larger amount of insanity than that of the present day" [133–136].

It was not only medical men who were alarmed by the rising insanity but the general public as well. Gossip and newspaper accounts of mad persons became commonplace, as one account in *The Times* describing the "Conduct of a Lunatic in a Church," in which a man "got into the pulpit just as the clergyman was coming from the vestry to read his sermon. . . . The man clung to the gas fittings and was not removed until after a desperate struggle with the sexton and his assistants." Such public accounts often included serious misdeeds, including one under a headline of "Horrible Circumstance," in which a "maniac" named Big Hector "lately visited Edderton, in the eastern portion of this county, where, having taken hold of a child (a girl), he ate the flesh off her arm, and the poor sufferer when relieved was, and still is, in a very painful and dangerous condition." By the end of the 1850s, one journal lamented "such a period as the present, when lunacy and lunatic affairs claim so large an amount of attention and interest on the part of the general public" [137–139].

In response to the rising alarm among the general public about the conditions of the asylums and the steadily increasing number of mad people, parliament in 1859 appointed yet another Select Committee on lunatics to investigate the situation. Testimony before the committee included a description of an asylum at London's Colney Hatch, which had opened in 1851 with accommodations for 1,220 "lunatic poor" but which "almost immediately . . . was filled with a mass of chronic patients." "And now," the testimony continued, "within a period of five years, it has again become necessary to appeal to the county to provide further accommodation for its pauper lunatics" [140].

5.8 Official Denial of the Problem

From 1859 onward the official position of the British government, as represented by the Lunacy Commission, was that insanity was not increasing. The "apparent" increases were said to be due to improved case finding and the accumulation of chronic cases in the asylums. Once established, this official position never changed. Year after year the Lunacy Commission's annual report listed increases in the number of insane persons in England, followed immediately by ritual assurances that the increases were only "apparent" due to an "accumulation" of cases.

The government's efforts to persuade the public that insanity was not increasing were helped immensely by England's psychiatric establishment. In 1841, physicians working in the asylums had organized the Association of Medical Officers of Asylums and Hospitals for the Insane, which later became the Medico-Psychological Association and eventually the Royal College of Psychiatrists. In 1853 this organization began publishing the *Journal of Mental Science*, later to become the *British Journal of Psychiatry*, regarded as the official voice of English psychiatry. From the beginning of its publication until 1895, the *Journal of Mental Science* was edited or coedited by four psychiatrists—John Bucknill, C. Lockhart Robertson, Henry Maudsley, and Hack Tuke—all of whom aggressively promoted the idea that insanity was not increasing. Thus, the official government position and the official psychiatric position reinforced and supported each other, and no matter how alarming the reported increases of insane persons, the increases were invariably labeled as being merely "apparent."

John Bucknill was superintendent of the Devonshire Asylum from 1844 to 1862. In 1853 he became the first editor of the *Journal of Mental Science* and later became president of the Medico-Psychological Association and was knighted. In an 1858 textbook written with Hack Tuke, he said:

> "On no subject has there been more absurd and illogical reasoning, or more hasty generalisations, than on the proportion of the insane to the population. . . . Highly important inferences are drawn with the utmost complacency, and apparently in entire ignorance of the fallacy which underlies such loose and worthless calculations. . . . In our own country there are two reasons why the proportion of the insane to the population appears to be greater than was formerly the case. The first is, that the disease is recognised as such to a far greater extent than formerly; and the second is, that we know, to a much greater extent than heretofore, the number of the insane throughout the country. In the short period of nineteen years, the estimated proportion of the insane in England rose from 1 in 7,300 to 1 in 769; a difference which led to the belief in the frightful increase of insanity, but which by no means warranted such a conclusion. The knowledge of an evil, and the existence of that evil, are two widely different things."

Bucknill also agreed with Lord Shaftesbury that if any portion of the "apparent" increase in insanity was real, that portion was probably attributable to "intemperance" and "the over-tasking of emotions" caused by advancing civilization [141].

In 1862 C. Lockhart Robertson assumed editorship of the *Journal of Mental Science*. Robertson was superintendent of the Sussex County Asylum from 1859 to 1870 and a president of the Medico-Psychological Association, and he labeled the increase of insanity in England as "a manifest fallacy." In 1869 he published a widely cited article entitled "The Alleged Increase of Lunacy," in which he acknowledged that there had been "an increase in the last twenty-five years in the number of registered lunatics of more than a hundred per cent," but he claimed that this was caused by better case finding, better statistics, and the accumulation of chronic cases in the asylums. He admitted that admissions to the asylums were still continuing to rise but said that this was no cause for concern since "the rate of increase is in a yearly decreasing ratio." He concluded that "the alleged increase of lunacy is a popular fallacy, unsupported by recent statistics" [142].

Robertson used the *Journal of Mental Science* as a forum to vigorously publicize his position. Summaries of his article "The Alleged Increase of Lunacy" were also published in popular periodicals, including *The Pall Mall Gazette*, the *Saturday Review*, and the *North British Review*, and Robertson dutifully reprinted these summaries in the *Journal of Mental Science*. In an 1871 issue, Robertson included a "Report on Insanity in Wiltshire," in which the author concluded that "the supposed increased liability to insanity in England at the present time, as compared with the earlier part of the century, may to a great extent, or even altogether, be imaginary, when the increase in the general population is considered." At the same time, Robertson continually reminded readers of the great advances being made by modern psychiatric treatments. In view of these advances, an increase in insanity was, in Robertson's view, a "terrible possibility which I entirely dispute" [143–145].

Following the 1859 Select Committee hearings, it became apparent that there still was much public concern about the rising insanity. According to Andrew Scull,

"The progressive increase in insanity was obvious to those with only the most casual acquaintance with the subject…Public fear of the legions of crazy men and women that society was apparently spawning at times verged on panic." To allay such fears, the Lunacy Commission increased the frequency of the census of insane persons to annually. The result reassured nobody. Year after year the result was more insane persons than the year before. Over the next 12 years, from 1860 to 1871, the total number of insane persons increased from 36,762 to 56,755, a 54 percent increase. When considering the growth of the general population, the increase was still a 33 percent increase, from 1.87 insane persons per 1,000 population to 2.49 per 1,000. Including the growth of population, there were three times more insane people in England in 1871 than there had been in 1829 [146].

Each year the new figures were announced, followed by predictable reassurances by the psychiatric establishment that the increase was only "apparent." The new cases had been there all along, they argued, and the ability to identify and count them had improved. The increase was thus merely a statistical artifact, nothing to worry about.

Most people were not reassured. In 1864 *The Times* noted: "Our asylums, private and public, now contain nearly twice as many patients as they did 15 years ago. . . . But this large number does not fully represent the total amount of insanity existing in the country; there are also the insane in gaols, the Chancery patients living out of asylums, and cases kept out of view for private or other reasons." In 1868 *The Times* reported that in the previous 10 years insane persons had increased "45 percent while the population is estimated to have increased rather more than 11 percent." The following year the *North British Review*, examining the statistics on insanity, concluded: "If we examine the effect of this at the end of a long series of years, we have a result which cannot fail to startle." And a few years later, *The Times* quoted a magistrate as saying that "if the lunacy continued to increase as at present, the insane would be in the majority and, freeing themselves, would put the sane in the asylums" [147, 148].

In 1870, Henry Maudsley followed doctors Bucknill and Robertson as the editor of the *Journal of Mental Science*. Although only 35 years old, he had already published a widely read textbook on *The Physiology and Pathology of the Mind*, had been nominated as president of the Medico-Psychological Association, and "had established himself by most measures as the dominant voice in the [psychiatric] profession." The fact that he had married the daughter of John Conolly, the most influential psychiatrist of the mid-nineteenth century, also was useful for Maudsley's career prospects. Although in later years Maudsley would distance himself from his psychiatric colleagues, in 1870, he was most interested in promoting his profession and himself [149].

It was at this time that Maudsley published the first of two articles in which he hoped to definitively discredit the idea that insanity was increasing. He argued that the claim "that so many more persons should be yearly going mad now than twenty-five years ago, seem to me a superstition which is, I will not say preposterous, but is certainly not probable in itself and not supported by facts." Using his considerable analytic and writing skills, Maudsley suggested four reasons why insanity only appeared to be increasing [150].

The first reason was the one that had been invoked by other critics of increasing insanity for many years—the closet theory. That is, that England had always had this number of insane persons, but they were "kept at home, or farmed out to their relatives, or taken care of in some other way of which there was no official knowledge." It was only when the asylums were built, claimed Maudsley, that these people appeared. The major problem with this argument was determining cause and effect: did the building of asylums bring existing insane persons out of the closet or did increasing insane persons appear thereby creating the need to build more asylums? And assuming that there was at least some truth to the closet theory, is it reasonable to expect this backlog of cases to continue appearing for half a century? Wouldn't you expect that at some point all the closets would have been emptied? In fact, Maudsley discussed this issue and predicted that all the old cases would be taken care of by 1883. As will become evident, that did not happen [151].

The second reason cited by Maudsley for why insanity was not really increasing was a broadening of the diagnostic categories. As he phrased it, "certain patients were registered as lunatics then who…would not have been classed as lunatics a quarter of a century before." Maudsley offered no supporting data, and in fact the reports of the Lunacy Commission contradicted him. For the last half of the nineteenth century, the diagnoses of patients were remarkably consistent; most of them were labeled with mania, melancholy, and dementia and a smaller number with general paralysis of the insane (brain syphilis), epileptic psychosis, and alcoholic insanity. Some asylum superintendents also contradicted Maudsley. The head of the Staffordshire Asylum, for example, said that his admission statistics "do not lend support to the idea which one hears expressed from time to time that many people are sent to asylums who have no business there. Such is certainly not our experience; on the contrary, we find that patients are frequently not brought here until it is impossible to keep them outside" [151, 152].

In more recent years, the question of broadened diagnostic categories as an explanation for the increasing insanity in England has been examined systematically. Psychiatric records from nineteenth-century asylums have been rediagnosed using modern diagnostic criteria. For example, a comparison of all admissions to Lancashire's Rainhill Asylum in 1890 and 1990, using the International Classification of Diseases (ICD 9), reported the following diagnostic breakdown:

	1890 admissions	1990 admissions
Psychoses (schizophrenia, manic-depressive illness, psychotic depression, hypomania, manic episode)	33%	40%
Depression	18%	24%
Drug-induced psychosis	0%	2%
Alcohol-related illness	8%	16%
Dementia (Alzheimer's and other)	6%	1%
Epilepsy	6%	0%
General paralysis of the insane	11%	0%
Mental subnormality	11%	0%
Acute confusional state	3%	2%
Anxiety-related illness	0%	5%
Personality disorder	0%	6%
No mental illness	4%	3%

Such results lend no support to the belief that patients admitted in 1890 were mild cases. These findings are also consistent with retrospective diagnostic studies of patients from nineteenth-century private asylums, including Trevor Turner's study of Ticehurst Asylum, Edward Renvoize and Allan Beveridge's study of the York Retreat, Franklin Klaf and John Hamilton's study of Bethlem Hospital, and William Parry-Jones's study of Duddeston Hall and Brislington House [153–157].

A "lower percentage of recoveries" was the third reason listed by Maudsley to explain the apparent increase in insanity. There is some evidence to support the fact that recovery rates for hospitalized persons decreased in the second half of the nineteenth century, including studies of the asylums at Lancashire, Buckinghamshire, Colney Hatch, and Hook Norton. Such findings were cited in 1890 as evidence that "the form of insanity was worse" than it had been earlier in the century. These findings are consistent with Robert Wilkins's findings of an increasing number of young patients admitted to Bethlem with symptoms of auditory and visual hallucinations between 1830 and 1899. It is also consistent with Hack Tuke's 1892 observation that "a large number of cases of pubescent and adolescent insanity terminate more unfavorably than the mental physician, guided in his prognosis by the general truth, has been led to expect." Such patients would now be diagnosed as having schizophrenia. It should also be noted that insofar as more severe cases were being seen with fewer recoveries as the nineteenth century progressed, this directly contradicts the claim that less severe cases were being hospitalized during those years [158, 159].

Finally, Maudsley argued that there was an apparent increase in insanity because insane persons were living longer "in well-conducted asylums where they are well fed, well clothed, and well housed." As evidence he cited three asylums in which patients were well fed as having a lower annual mortality rate compared to four asylums in which patients were not as well fed with higher mortality rates. In fact, however, asylum death rates varied widely by year and by asylum. Infectious diseases such as typhus, cholera, pneumonia, tuberculosis, and syphilis were the most common causes of death in the asylums, followed by cardiovascular diseases. Given the actual conditions of most of the public asylums, it is likely that insane persons who entered asylums lived shorter lives, not longer lives, than if they had remained living in the community.   This possibility had been suggested as early as 1835 by William Farr who calculated that death rates in asylums were three to six times greater than that of the general population at comparable age levels, and these figures were confirmed in 1879. For patients ages 20 to 24, the Lunacy Commission reported in 1906 that "the insane death-rate is nearly twenty times that of the general death-rate." However, given the epidemics of infectious diseases that frequently devastated the overcrowded asylums (e.g., cholera in 1832–1833 killed up to 49 percent of the asylum inmates), one can argue that increasing institutionalization of insane persons in the nineteenth century may have ultimately decreased their total number by killing larger numbers than would have died had they been living in the community. Thus by increasing the death rate of insane persons, the asylums may have decreased the rate of rising insanity, not increased it as Maudsley claimed [160–162].

By the late 1870s, Henry Maudsley "had established himself as the preeminent figure among British alienists" and he remained so until his death in 1918. Since Maudsley had said that the increasing insanity was not real but only apparent, that would be the official position of the psychiatrists. Hack Tuke, who followed Maudsley as the editor of *Journal of Mental Science* from 1880 until 1895, illustrated this position. Andrew Scull has labeled Tuke "the most unembarrassed apologist for Victorian asylumdom." William Bynum characterized Tuke as "a good 'party' man, devoted to improving the status of his profession in Britain." For example, in his *Chapters in the History of the Insane in the British Isles*, Tuke claimed "remarkable progress effected in the asylum care of our lunacy population." Although early in his career Tuke had expressed uncertainty about whether insanity was increasing or not, he later concluded that "the increase of insanity is apparent rather than real, being mainly due to accumulation" [163–167].

Tuke wrote extensively about the alleged increase of insanity and analyzed the available statistics from the Lunacy Commission to try to prove his point. He advocated the use of first admissions, rather than the total patients hospitalized, as "the only sound test of the increase of insanity." For example, in 1882, he recorded the first admissions per 10,000 total population for 12 years as follows:

1869	4.71	1875	5.19
1870	4.54	1876	5.30
1871	4.62	1877	5.28
1872	4.59	1878	5.36
1873	4.80	1879	5.20
1874	5.03	1880	5.19

His conclusion was that "the ratio of the yearly increase of the fresh admissions to the population has been slight," when in fact the increase was 10 percent over the 12-year period. By 1894 first admissions per population had increased another 10 percent; Tuke dismissed the figures, saying: "I have now reason to believe that the returns which have been since published [since 1880] cannot be trusted" [168].

For a "good 'party' man" like Hack Tuke, increasing insanity was simply unacceptable, as it had been for Bucknill, Robertson, and Maudsley before him. Tuke labeled the idea that insanity was increasing "a melancholy theory" that "would unsettle our belief in the onward progress of mankind, it would shake the very foundation of our faith." Increasing insanity would imply not only that the asylums had failed but also that the psychiatrists themselves had failed. It was an unacceptable possibility. As Mr. Podsnap said in Dickens's *Our Mutual Friend*, "I don't want to know about it; I don't want to discuss it; I don't want to admit it!" [169, 170]

Despite the assurances that improvement in asylum conditions had been "well nigh incredible" and Hack Tuke's claims of "remarkable progress," the continuing influx of insane individuals in the closing years of the nineteenth century overwhelmed the asylums. In 1824 there had been only eight public asylums with an average size of 116 beds. By 1860 there were 41 asylums with an average of 386 beds and, by 1890, 66 asylums with an average of 802 beds. Each annual report of the Lunacy Commission reported new asylums under construction, new wings being added to existing asylums, and the conversion of "several houses on the estate lately occupied by attendants . . . being prepared for the reception of patients." The West Riding Asylum had opened in 1818 with 150 beds; by the end of the century, it had 1,469 beds, almost a tenfold increase. As early as 1856, John Bucknill, superintendent of the badly overcrowded Devonshire Asylum, boarded out "quiet, chronic, female patients in neighboring cottages beyond the asylum grounds" and rented "a house in the nearby seaside town of Exmouth, where he boarded forty to forty-five quiet female patients under the care of a resident medical officer . . . and two resident female nurses," harbingers of deinstitutionalization, which would come a century later [171–173].

5.9   The Debate Winds Down

Despite the constant assurances by some of the leaders of English psychiatry that insanity was not really increasing, most people, including most psychiatrists, believed that it was. James Crichton-Browne, superintendent of the Yorkshire West Riding Asylum, wrote: "It is impossible for us to acquiesce in the soothing doctrine now being disseminated that the alleged increase of lunacy is only a popular fallacy"; rather, he said, it was clear "that an actual as well as an apparent augmentation in the numbers of our insane poor is rapidly in progress." In a similar vein, Martin Duncan said that it was time "to admit that for once popular fallacy is supported by recent statistics. . . . There is a steady increase in the lunacy of the population of England, Wales, and Ireland. . . . Insanity remains as a dead-weight on the statistics of our social miseries." John Arlidge noted that "the increase of lunacy . . . [is] a painful and perplexing fact" and that available data "indisputably [point] to an absolutely increased production in the community." Harrington Tuke, not related to Hack Tuke, also claimed that "these figures would appear to prove that a great wave of insanity is slowly advancing, but making each year a definite progress." And Robert Jamieson of the Royal Aberdeen Hospital claimed that "the most remarkable phenomenon of our time has been the alarming increase of insanity" [174–176].

As the century drew to a close, the leadership of English psychiatry decided to try once again to counter the public alarm about rising insanity by holding a "special enquiry into the alleged increase of insanity in England and Wales" under the commissioners in lunacy. Because the commissioners had had primary responsibility for the problem of insanity since 1845 and had stated many times that insanity was not increasing, the outcome of the enquiry was a foregone conclusion.

The resulting "Special Report on the Alleged Increase of Insanity" was published in 1897. Large portions appear to have been adapted from an 1890 study by Noel Humphreys, a statistician, who had concluded:

> Without therefore venturing to say that there has been no increase of insanity in England in recent years, many reasons have been pointed out for refusing to accept any insanity statistics that we at present possess as conclusive evidence of a real increase of the rate of occurring insanity.

Humphreys' cautious conclusions were eagerly enlarged upon by some psychiatrists. George Savage said they put to rest "one of the bugbears of the age, the idea that insanity was running like wildfire through the whole population." Hack Tuke also "rejoiced to find the conclusions at which Mr. Humphreys had arrived were so much in accordance with what might be regarded as an encouraging and satisfactory mode of viewing the great question of the alleged increase of insanity in England and Wales" [177].

The 1897 Special Report included data on the increase in asylum patients between 1859 and 1896. Especially damning was a table showing that first admissions had increased from 4.71 per 10,000 total population in 1869 to 5.16 in 1879, 5.29 in 1889, and 6.09 in 1895. The report acknowledged that "the upward progress ... of first attacks out of proportion to population seems *prima facie* to indicate the increase of insanity which has been alleged, and we must now inquire if there are any circumstances which modify its apparently significant influence" [178].

The bulk of the 1897 *Special Report* then examined in great detail the same reasons why insanity was not increasing that had been invoked by Henry Maudsley in the 1870s. First, most insane persons had been kept at home and only became recognized when the asylums were built. Second, the diagnostic category of insanity had been broadened, thus bringing less severely ill individuals to the asylums. Third, over the course of the nineteenth century, fewer patients were recovering, thus decreasing discharges and increasing the census. And, finally, insane persons were living longer in the asylums than they would have if they had remained at home.

In fact, the data cited by the 1897 Special Report was no more convincing than it had been 20 years earlier when offered by Maudsley. The only explanation for which there was evidence—that insanity was clinically becoming more severe in the nineteenth century—was hardly one that would have reassured the press or the public regarding their fears of rising insanity. The commissioners concluded their report by stating that "we have been unable to satisfy ourselves that there has been any important increase of occurring or fresh insanity." Given their own data, such a conclusion was wishful thinking.

Five months following the publication of the 1897 Special Report, the commissioners in lunacy issued their annual report for 1897, showing a total of 99,365 insane persons, an increase of 2,919 since the previous year, the increase being "the largest on record." The following year, the total increased by an additional 2,607 patients to 101,972, which the commissioners labeled "this huge mass of insane humanity." The figures appeared to be an additional refutation of their 1897 report [179, 180].

Nor was the English press convinced by the 1897 Special Report. The *Westminster Review* labeled it "ridiculous efforts to gloss over and explain away undeniable facts. ... That there is an actual increase is indubitable, notwithstanding the dogmatic but puerile asseverations of the Commissioners in Lunacy to the contrary. ... Were the Commissioners in Lunacy cross-examined on their own figures and the inferences they have drawn, a lamentable appearance might be predicted" [181].

The most damning criticism of the English Lunacy Commission, however, came from W. J. Corbet, the chief clerk of the Irish Lunacy Department and a former member of parliament from Ireland. He said the authors of the special report had "devoted all their energies to combating the idea that insanity is on the increase. . . . a more remarkable composition has rarely, if ever, emanated from official brain or pen." Not a man to hide his opinions, Corbet had previously accused the commissioners of "fossilized officialism" as well as "Lilliputian logic" and had compared them to "simple parents fondling their deformed offspring . . . hugging the fallacy they have themselves created, until, by constant repetition, they at length evidently believe in the soundness of their conclusions, though the figures given in their own reports are convincing to the contrary" [182].

Following the publication of the 1897 Special Report, public discussion of increasing insanity in England continued for another decade, as the number of institutionalized insane increased from 101,972 (3.24 per 1,000) in 1898 to 126,084 (3.60 per 1,000) in 1908. Newspapers continued to express concern about "the grave increase of lunacy. . . . Assuming a similar increase in the future, what is the outlook for, say, 50 years hence?" And the psychiatric establishment continued to offer a multitude of reasons to explain why the increase was not real but merely apparent, as in this 1903 report: "The question that at once presents itself is whether this growing ratio means that insanity on the whole is increasing. There are several other explanations which would require to be borne in mind before admitting such an unpleasant one" [183].

It is important to understand how dissonant the idea of rising insanity was at the end of the Victorian era. England had become *the* dominant world power. It had assumed, in Kipling's phrase, "the white man's burden" and had overrun, annexed, or purchased one quarter of the earth's land surface. England controlled territory from the Transvaal to Cyprus and Uganda to Fiji, had purchased the Suez Canal, and had proclaimed Queen Victoria as the Empress of India. By 1892 "Britain had more registered shipping tonnage than the rest of the world put together." At home, "the horsepower used in British industry increased from two million in 1870 to ten million in 1907." Benjamin Disraeli described England as having undergone a "convulsion of prosperity." However, amid this prosperity, the number of insane persons had risen from 8,941 in 1829 to 126,084 in 1908, more than quadrupling the number even when the increase in population was taken into account. Worse yet, visitors from France, America, and other countries had publicly commented on the problem. Insanity was an uninvited and most unwelcome guest at England's celebratory banquet. A solution to the problem would come from unexpected events [184].

Even the psychiatrists were trying to solve the problem of increasing insanity; political events were taking place in Europe that would soon focus England's attention on other problems. In Hamburg the kaiser asserted Germany's "place in the sun" and renewed his nation's alliance with Austria and Italy. The Balkan Wars spread unrest progressively across Europe. Finally, on June 28, 1914, Archduke Franz Ferdinand, heir to the Austrian throne, was assassinated in Sarajevo, and within weeks, Europe was at war.

World War I substantially altered the perception of insanity in England, reducing it from a growing threat to merely an ongoing inconvenience. Insanity was no longer viewed as an increasing affliction of the body politic, evoking letters in *The*

Times, but instead as a chronic blemish on the human condition for which little could be done. The pervasive nineteenth-century fear that insanity was increasing was largely eclipsed by current events.

In 1914, when the war began, there were 138,055 insane persons in 97 English asylums. By January, 1915, the number had climbed to 140,466, or a rate of 3.98 per 1,000 total population. This contrasts with the first reliable national census in 1829 which counted 8,941 insane persons or 0.79 per 1,000 population (Fig. 5.3). Over the 86-year period, between 1829 and 1915, there was therefore a fivefold increase in the number of insane persons per population. One out of every 250 persons of all ages was confined to an insane asylum, and among young adults, the rate was much higher.

World War I had a direct effect on the asylums because hospitals were needed to treat large number of war casualties. Therefore, the government "took over a number of county asylums, and other asylums had to accept and house their displaced patients for the duration of the war." Insane patients who were less severely disabled were sent home, many new admissions were refused, and in the remaining asylums "extra beds were squeezed into the dormitories, the corridors [were] filled with beds, [and] other rooms were converted into bedrooms." In addition, almost half of the medical and nursing staff went off to fight, and food rations for the mental hospitals were reduced [185].

Then, at the height of this crowding, understaffing, and reduced food rations, the influenza pandemic arrived. The death rate among patients soared, as can be seen from the deaths in the Buckinghamshire Asylum:

1910–1914:	67	average for each year
1915:	81	
1916:	110	
1917:	129	
1918:	257	

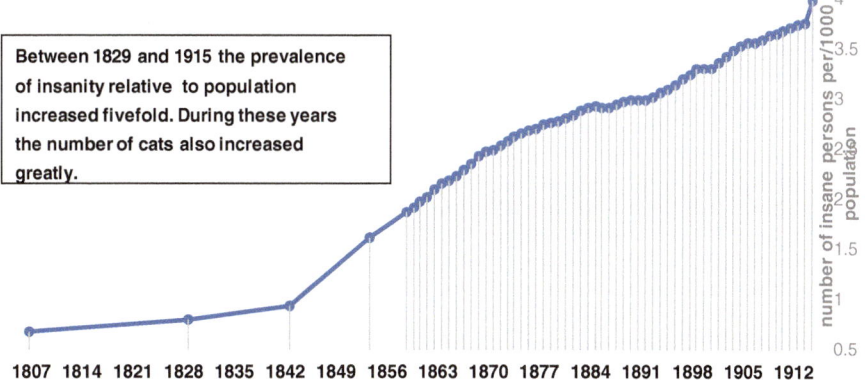

Between 1829 and 1915 the prevalence of insanity relative to population increased fivefold. During these years the number of cats also increased greatly.

Fig. 5.3 Number of insane persons per 1,000 population, England and Wales. (Source of data: E. Fuller Torrey and Judy Miller, The Invisible Plague. Table 1. pages 345–346.)

In 1918, almost one third of all the patients died in this asylum. Nationally, the total number of 1918 asylum deaths was 19,515, double the prewar rate. By 1920, then, the census of England's mental hospitals had been reduced 17 percent to 116,764. After a century of looking for a solution to the increasing insanity, two had finally emerged—war and influenza [186].

References

1. Macalpine I, Hunter R. George III and the mad business. London: Pimlico; 1991. p. 291.
2. Tague, IH. Animal companions: Pets and social change in 18th century Britain. University Park Pennsylvania: Pennsylvania State University Press; 2015. p. 2.
3. Ritvo H. The animal estate. Cambridge: Harvard University Press; 1987. p. 86.
4. Keenan S. Animals in the house. New York: Scholastic; 2007. p. 30.
5. Rogers, KM. Cat. London: Reaktion Books; 2006. p. 47.
6. Amato S. Beastly possessions. Toronto: University of Toronto Press; 2015. p. 29.
7. Vocelle LA. Revered and reviled: a complete history of the domestic cat. Great Cat Publications, 2016. [no city listed]. p. 262.
8. Murfin L. Popular leisure in the lake counties. Manchester: Manchester University Press; 1990. p. 14.
9. Rush W. Thoughts on insanity. Knick. 1836;7:33–6.
10. Amato S. Beastly possessions. Toronto: University of Toronto Press; 2015. p. 63.
11. Entry for Robert Southey on Wikipedia.
12. Winslow HM, Concerning cats. Boston; Lothrop Publishing, 1900. p. 112.
13. Winslow HM, Concerning cats. Boston: Lothrop Publishing; 1900. p. 112.
14. Jamison KR, Touched with fire: Manic-depressive illness and the artistic temperment. New York: Free Press; 1993. p. 169.
15. Rogers, KM. Cat. London: Reaktion Books; 2006. p. 62.
16. Vocelle LA. Revered and reviled: a complete history of the domestic cat. Great Cat Publications, 2016. [no city listed]. p. 289.
17. Ackroyd P. Blake. London: Vintage; 1995. p. 235.
18. Rogers, KM. Cat. London: Reaktion Books; 2006. p. 94.
19. Vocelle LA. Revered and reviled: a complete history of the domestic cat. Great Cat Publications, 2016. [no city listed]. p. 309.
20. Rogers, KM. Cat. London: Reaktion Books; 2006. p. 90, 63.
21. Ritvo H. The animal estate. Cambridge: Harvard University Press; 1987. p. 129.
22. Winslow HM, Concerning cats. Boston: Lothrop Publishing; 1900. p. 128,114.
23. Vocelle LA. Revered and reviled: a complete history of the domestic cat. Great Cat Publications, 2016. [no city listed], 315.
24. Anonymous, "The cat about town," Living age 217: 47–49, April–June 1898.
25. Champfleury M. The cat past and present. London: George Bell; 1885. p. 64.
26. Winslow HM, Concerning cats. Boston: Lothrop Publishing; 1900. p. 119–120.
27. Amato S. Beastly possessions. Toronto: University of Toronto Press; 2015. p. 10.
28. Lynnlee JL. Purrfection the cat. West Chester: Schiffer Publishing; 1990. p. 25–6.
29. Champfleury M. The cat past and present. London: George Bell; 1885. p. 22.
30. Champfleury M. The cat past and present. London: George Bell; 1885. p. 75.
31. Bugler, C. The Cat: 3,500 years of the cat in art. New York: Merrell; 2011. p. 248.
32. Pargeter W. Observations on maniacal disorders. London: Routledge; 1988. p. 1–3. Originally published in 1792
33. Leigh D. The historical development of British Psychiatry. Vol I. Oxford: Pergamon; 1961. p. 144.
34. Haslam J. Observations on insanity. London: F. and C. Rivington; 1798, Preface, iii.

35. Persaud RD. A comparison of symptoms recorded from the same patients by an asylum doctor and 'a constant observer' in 1823: the implications for theories about psychiatric illness in history. Hist Psychiatry. 1992;3:79–94.
36. Hare E. Was insanity on the increase? Br J Psychiatry. 1983;142:439–55, quoting Harper.
37. Carpenter PK. Descriptions of schizophrenia in the psychiatry of Georgian Britain: John Haslam and James Tilly Matthews. Compr Psychiatry. 1989;30:332–8.
38. Leigh D. The historical development of British Psychiatry. Vol I. Oxford: Pergamon; 1961. p. 122.
39. Cox J. Practical observations on insanity. London: Baldwin; 1804.
40. Stark W. Remarks on the construction of public hospitals for the cure of mental derangement. Edinburgh: Ballantyne; 1807.
41. Reid J. Report of diseases. Monthly Magazine. 25(1808):166, 374.
42. Byrd M. Visits to Bedlam: Madness in literature in the 18th century. Columbia: University of South Carolina Press. 1974. p. 128.
43. House of Commons, Report of the Select Committee on the State of Criminal and Pauper Lunatics, 1807.
44. Jones K. A history of the mental health services. London: Routledge and Kegan Paul; 1972. p. 58.
45. Powell R. Observations upon the comparative prevalence of insanity at different periods. Med Transact. 1813;4:131–59.
46. Smith LD. Cure, comfort and safe custody: public lunatic asylums in early nineteenth century England. London: Leicester University Press; 1999. p. 24.
47. Crammer J, A silent history: Buckinghamshire County Pauper Lunatic Asylum—St. John's. London: Gaskell, Royal College of Psychiatrists; 1990. p. 15.
48. Skultans V. English madness: ideas on insanity, 1580–1890. London: Routledge and Kegan Paul; 1979. p. 98.
49. Smith LD. Cure, comfort and safe custody: public lunatic asylums in early nineteenth century England. London: Leicester University Press; 1999. p. 39.
50. Smith LD. Cure, comfort and safe custody: public lunatic asylums in early nineteenth century England. London: Leicester University Press; 1999. p. 40–1.
51. Hare E. Was insanity on the increase? Br J Psychiatry. 1983;142:439–55, quoting Crowther.
52. Hill G. An essay on the prevention and cure of insanity. London: Longman, Hurst, Rees, Orme and Brown; 1814.
53. Simond L. An American in regency England. London: Robert Maxwell; 1815. p. 110, 115.
54. Arnold T. Observations on the nature, kinds, causes, and prevention of insanity, lunacy or madness. New York: Arno Press; 1976.; Originally published in 1782. p. 17–27.
55. Arnold T. Observations on the nature, kinds, causes, and prevention of insanity, lunacy or madness. New York: Arno Press; 1976.; Originally published in 1782. p. 26.
56. Rowley W. A treatise of female, nervous, hysterical, hypochondriacal, bilious, convulsive diseases. London: C. Nourse; 1788. p. 253–4.
57. Porter R, editor. The Faber book of madness. London: Faber and Faber; 1991. p. 120.
58. Scull A. The most solitary of afflictions. New Haven: Yale University Press; 1993. p. 157.
59. Porter R. Mind-forged manacles: A history of madness in England. Cambridge: Harvard University Press, 1987; p. 161.
60. Browne WAF. What asylums were, are, and ought to be. Edinburgh: Black; 1837; New York: Arno Press; 1976. p. 52.
61. Moore CA. Backgrounds of English literature. New York: Octagon books; 1969. p. 190.
62. Simond L. An American in regency England. London: Robert Maxwell; 1815. p. 110.
63. Browne WAF. What asylums were, are, and ought to be. Edinburgh: Black; 1837; New York: Arno Press; 1976. p. 61.
64. Scull A. The most solitary of afflictions. New Haven: Yale University Press; 1993. p. 158.
65. Pinel PA. Treatise on insanity. Sheffield: Todd; 1806. p. 114.
66. Courtney WF. Young Charles Lamb, 1775–1802. New York: New York University Press; 1982. p. 108, 110, quoting Lamb's letters to Coleridge.

67. Courtney WF. Young Charles Lamb, 1775–1802. New York: New York University Press; 1982. p. 114, 115.

68. Lucas EV, editor. The letters of Charles Lamb, vol. 3. New Haven: Yale University Press; 1935. p. 370, 417.

69. Lucas EV, editor. The letters of Charles Lamb, vol. 3. New Haven, Yale University Press; 1935. I, 9.

70. Jamison KR, Touched with fire: Manic-depressive illness and the artistic temperment. New York: Free Press; 1993. p 67, 221.

71. Faulkner TC, editor. Selected letters and journals of George Crabbe. Oxford: Clarendon Press; 1985. p. 102.

72. Shimer M. Madness and the muse in nineteenth-century English romantic poetry. Ann Arbor: UMI Dissertation Service; 1996. p. 73.

73. Shimer M. Madness and the muse in nineteenth-century English romantic poetry. Ann Arbor: UMI Dissertation Service; 1996. p. 127.

74. Youngquist P. Madness and Blake's myth. University Park: Pennsylvania State University Press; 1989. p. 3, 16, 105–107, 170n.

75. Ackroyd P. Blake. London: Vintage; 1995. p. 233.

76. Whitehead F. George Crabbe: a reappraisal. Selinsgrove: Susquehanna University Press; 1995. p. 50.

77. Pollard A, editor. Crabbe: the critical heritage. Boston: Routledge and Kegan Paul; 1972. p. 53, quoting the Oxford review, January 1808.

78. Whitehead F. Crabbe: a reappraisal. Selinsgrove: Susquehanna University Press; 1995. p. 143.

79. Shimer M. Madness and the muse in nineteenth-century English romantic poetry. Ann Arbor: UMI Dissertation Service; 1996. p. 200.

80. Jamison KR, Touched with fire: Manic-depressive illness and the artistic temperment. New York: Free Press; 1993. p. 179, 2, 43, 171.

81. Jamison KR, Touched with fire: Manic-depressive illness and the artistic temperment. New York: Free Press; 1993. p. 179, 69.

82. Jamison KR, Touched with fire: Manic-depressive illness and the artistic temperment. New York: Free Press; 1993. p. 67.

83. Oberhelman DD. Mad encounters: nineteenth-century British psychological medicine and the Victorian novel, 1840–1870. Ann Arbor: UMI Dissertation Services; 1993. p. 87.

84. Buck HM. Insanity, character roles, and authorial milieu: a study of madness in selected Waverley novels. Ann Arbor: UMI Dissertation Services; 1987. p. 30.

85. Claridge G, Pryor R, Watkins G. Sounds from the bell jar. New York: St. Martin's Press; 1990. p. 132–3.

86. Haughton H, editor. John Clare in context. Cambridge: Cambridge University Press; 1994. p. 10.

87. Quiller-Couch AT, editor. The Oxford book of English verse 1250–1900. Oxford: Clarendon Press; 1907.

88. Colley AC. Tennyson and madness. Athens: University of Georgia Press; 1983. p. 258, 266.

89. Bucknill JC. Maud and other poems, by Alfred Tennyson. Asylum J Ment Sci. 15 (1855): 94–104. Tennyson AL, The works of Tennyson, vol. 4, The Princess and Maud. New York: AMS Press; 1970. p. 209.

90. Bronte C. Jane Eyre. New York: Penguin Books; 1982. p. 295.

91. Small H. Love's madness: medicine, the novel, and female insanity, 1800–1865. Oxford: Clarendon Press; 1996. p. 165, quoting Bronte's letter of January 4, 1848.

92. Colley AC. Tennyson and madness. Athens: University of Georgia Press; 1983. p. 10.

93. Small H. Love's madness: medicine, the novel, and female insanity, 1800–1865. Oxford: Clarendon Press; 1996. p. 165, quoting Bronte's letter of January 28, 1848.

94. Mannheim L. Dickens' fools and madmen. Dickens Stud Ann. 1972;2:69–97.

95. Dickens C. The works of Charles Dickens: Pickwick papers, vol. 208. New York: Books, Inc; 1841.

96. Oberhelman DD. Mad encounters: nineteenth-century British psychological medicine and the Victorian novel, 1840–1870. Ann Arbor: UMI Dissertation Services; 1993. p. 381, 393, 389.
97. The works of Charles Dickens: Barnaby Rudge. New York: Books, Inc.; 1841. p. 521.
98. Dickens C. A curious dance. Household Words. January 17, 1852.
99. Dickens C, Collins W. The lazy tour of two idle apprentices. In: Seaside library, vol. XIX, no. 372. New York: George Munro; 1857.
100. Oberhelman DD. Mad encounters: nineteenth-century British psychological medicine and the Victorian novel, 1840–1870. Ann Arbor: UMI Dissertation Services; 1993. p. 132–3.
101. Oberhelman DD. Mad encounters: nineteenth-century British psychological medicine and the Victorian novel, 1840–1870. Ann Arbor: UMI Dissertation Services; 1993. p. 126–127, 179, 198.
102. Skilton D. Introduction to Lady Audley's secret, by Mary Elizabeth Braddon. Oxford: Oxford University Press; 1987.
103. Braddon ME. Lady Audley's secret. Harmondsworth: Penguin; 1985. p. 293.
104. Entries on Wikipedia for John Robert Cozene, Lemuel Abbott, James Gillray, and Richard Dadd.
105. Scull A, et al. Masters of bedlam. Princeton: Princeton University Press; 1996. p. 97.
106. Burrows GM. Commentaries on the causes, forms, symptoms, and treatment, moral and medical, of insanity. New York: Arno Press; 1976.; Originally published in 1828. p. 81.
107. Burrows GM. An inquiry into certain errors relative to insanity. London: Underwood; 1820. p. 54.
108. Burrows GM. An inquiry into certain errors relative to insanity. London: Underwood; 1820. p. 80, 81, 83.
109. Macalpine I, Hunter R. George III and the Mad Business. London: Pimlico; 1991. p. 294.
110. Anonymous. Inquiries relative to insanity. Q Rev. 24(1821):181.
111. Anonymous. Insanity. Q Rev. 1830;42:351–77.
112. Halliday A. A report on the number of lunatics and idiots in England and Wales. In: A letter to Lord Robert Seymour. London: Underwood; 1829.
113. Halliday A. A general view of the present state of lunatics, and lunatic asylums. London: Underwood; 1828. p. 80.
114. Prichard J. A treatise on insanity and other disorders affecting the mind. London: Sherwood, Gilbert and Piper; 1835. p. 350.
115. Scull A, et al. Masters of bedlam. Princeton: Princeton University Press; 1996. p. 89, 97, 103.
116. Report of the metropolitan commissioners in lunacy to the Lord Chancellor. London: Bradbury and Evans; 1844. Appendix F.
117. Jones K. A history of the mental health services. London: Routledge and Kegan Paul; 1972. p. 227.
118. Smith LD. Cure, comfort and safe custody: public lunatic asylums in early nineteenth century England. London: Leicester University Press; 1999. p. 176–7.
119. Parry-Jones W. The trade in Lunacy: a study of the private madhouses in England in the 18th and 19th centuries. London: Routledge and Kegan Paul; 1972; p. 65.
120. Colley AC. Tennyson and madness. Athens: University of Georgia Press; 1983. p. 12.
121. Scull A. Psychiatrists and historical 'facts': part two: re-writing the history of asylumdom. Hist Psychiatry. 1995;6:387–94.
122. Jones K. A history of the mental health services. London: Routledge and Kegan Paul; 1972. p. 89.
123. Walton JK. Casting out and bringing back in Victorian England: pauper lunatics, 1840–1870. In: Bynum et al. Anatomy of madness, vol. 2. p. 132.
124. Hare E. Was insanity on the increase? Br J Psychiatry. 1983;142: 439–55, quoting John Arledge.
125. Scull A. The most solitary of afflictions. New Haven: Yale University Press; 1993. p. 268, note 2.
126. Crammer J. Asylum history. London: Gaskell; 1990. p. 38–9.

127. Haguch. Comments on the report of the commissioners in lunacy and the swing of the pendulum. Westminster Rev. 1897;148:672–81.
128. Ayers GM. England's first state hospitals and the metropolitan asylums board, 1867–1930. London: Wellcome Institute; 1971. p. 38.
129. Jones K. A history of the mental health services. London: Routledge and Kegan Paul; 1972. p. 124.
130. McCandless P. 'Build! Build!': The controversy over the care of the chronically insane in England, 1855–1870. Bull Hist Med. 1979;53:553–74.
131. Hodgkinson, "Provision for pauper lunatics."
132. Scull A. The most solitary of afflictions. New Haven: Yale University Press; 1993. p. 160.
133. Burnett CM. Insanity tested by science. London: Highley; 1848.
134. Anonymous. Familiar views of lunacy and lunatic life. London: Parker; 1850. p. 101–2.
135. Maddox AB. Practical observations on nervous and mental disorders. London: Simpkin, Marshall; 1854. p. 13.
136. Hawkes J. On the increase of insanity. J Psychol Med Mental Pathol. 1857;10:508–21.
137. The Times, August 6, 1850, 5 f.
138. "Horrible Circumstance": The Times, October 7, 1844, 4 f.
139. Anonymous. 13th Report of the commission on lunacy. J Ment Sci. 1860;6:141–56.
140. Report of the Select Committee, 1859, Appendix 7, 324, quoted in W. J. Corbet. The holocaust at Colney Hatch. Westminster Rev. 159(1903):383–93.
141. Bucknill JC, Tuke DH. A manual of psychological medicine. London: Churchill; 1858. p. 32, 108.
142. Robertson CL. Lunacy in England. J Psychol Med Ment Pathol. 7(1881):185–6. The alleged increase of lunacy. J Ment Sci. 15(1869):1–23.
143. Journal of Mental Science 15 (1869):317–318, 446–447.
144. Journal of Mental Science 16 (1871):481, 492.
145. Robertson CL. Lunacy in England. J Psychol Med Ment Pathol. 7(1881):185–6. The alleged increase of lunacy. J Ment Sci. 15(1869):1–23.
146. Scull A. The most solitary of afflictions. New Haven: Yale University Press; 1993. p. 337–8.
147. The Times. January 11, 1860; August 2, 1868. April. June 30, 1864;5:1877.
148. Anonymous. The increase in lunacy. North Br Rev. 50(1869):123.
149. Scull A, et al. Masters of bedlam. Princeton: Princeton University Press; 1996. p. 233.
150. Maudsley H. Is insanity on the increase? Br Med J. 1872;1:36–9.
151. Maudsley H. The alleged increase of insanity. J Ment Sci. 1877;23:45–54.
152. Asylum reports. J Ment Sci. 44(1898):195.
153. Parker RR, et al. County of Lancaster Asylum, Rainhill: 100 years ago and now. Hist Psychiatry. 1993;4:95–105.
154. Turner T. Rich and mad in Victorian England. Psychol Med. 1989;19:29–44.
155. Renvoize EB, Beveridge AW. Mental illness and the late Victorians: a study of patients admitted to three asylums in York, 1880–1884. Psychol Med. 1989;19:19–28.
156. Klaf F, Hamilton J. Schizophrenia—a hundred years ago and today. J Ment Sci. 1961;107:819–27.
157. Parry-Jones W. The trade in Lunacy: a study of the private madhouses in England in the 18th and 19th centuries. London: Routledge and Kegan Paul; 1972. p. 328–330.
158. Wilkins R. Hallucinations in children and teenagers admitted to Bethlem Royal Hospital in the nineteenth century and their possible relevance to the incidence of schizophrenia. J Child Psychol Psychiatry. 1987;28:569–80.
159. Tuke DH. A dictionary of psychological medicine. Philadelphia: Blakiston; 1892.
160. Mitchell A. Contribution to the study of death rates of persons in asylums. J Ment Sci. 1879;25:1–4.
161. Lunacy commission report. J Ment Sci. 52(1906):142–7.
162. Walton J. The treatment of pauper lunatics in Victorian England: the case of Lancaster asylum 1816–70. In: Scull A, editor. Madhouses, mad-doctors, and madmen: the social history of psychiatry in the Victorian era. Philadelphia: University of Pennsylvania Press; 1981. p. 171.

163. Scull A, et al. Masters of bedlam. Princeton: Princeton University Press; 1996. p. 234.
164. Scull A. The most solitary of afflictions. New Haven: Yale University Press; 1993. p. 325.
165. Bynum WF. Tuke's dictionary and psychiatry at the turn of the century. In: Berrios GE and Freeman H, 150 Years of British Psychiatry, 1841–1991. London: Royal College of Psychiatrists; 1991. p. 164.
166. Tuke DH. Alleged increase of insanity. J Ment Sci. 1894;40:219–31.
167. Tuke DH. Chapters in the history of the insane in the British isles. London: Kegan Paul, Trench; 1882. p. 261.
168. Tuke DH. Alleged increase of insanity. J Ment Sci. 1894;40:219–31. Tuke DH. Chaptes in the history of the insane in the British isles. London: Kegan Paul, Trench; 1882. Hare E. Was insanity on the increase? Br J Psychiatry. 1983;142.
169. Psychological retrospect. Am J Insanity. 30(1874):476–7. Tuke H. Presidential address. J Ment Sci. 19(1873):327–40 and 479–85.
170. The works of Charles Dickens: our mutual friend. New York: Books, Inc.; 1841. p. 130.
171. Jones K. Lunacy, law and conscience 1744–1845. London: Routledge and Kegan Paul; 1955. p. 116.
172. Lunacy Commission reports: "Lunacy in England," The Times, January 4, 1878, 6 f. Allderidge P. Hospitals, madhouses and asylums. Brit J Psychiatry. 1999;134:321–34.
173. Scull A. The most solitary of afflictions. New Haven: Yale University Press; 1993. p. 209.
174. Robertson CL. A further note on the alleged increase of insanity. J Ment Sci. 1871;16:473–97.
175. Duncan PM. On insanity. J Sci. 1870;7:165–86.
176. Hare E. Was insanity on the increase? Br J Psychiatry. 1983;142:439–55.
177. Humphreys NA. Statistics of insanity in England. J R Stat Soc. 1890;53:201–52.
178. Special report on the alleged increase of insanity. 1897, 16.
179. J Ment Sci. 44(1898):113–26.
180. J Ment Sci. 45(1899):139–48.
181. Haguch. Comments on the report of the commissioners in lunacy and the swing of the pendulum. Westminster Rev. 1897;148:672–81.
182. Corbet WJ. Plain speaking about lunacy. Westminster Rev. 148(1897):117–25; The increase of insanity. 1896; The increase of insanity. Fortnightly Rev. 59 (n.s. 53) (1893):7–19.
183. The Times, August 28, 1903, 7 f. "56th Report," J MentaSci. 49(1903):126.
184. Briggs A. A social history of England. New York: Penguin; 1999. p. 216, 245.
185. Crammer J. Asylum history. London: Gaskell; 1990. p. 75.
186. Crammer J. Asylum history. London: Gaskell; 1990. p. 77.

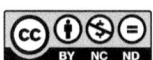

Additional Links Between Toxoplasmosis and Psychosis

6.1 Survey of the Historical Data

After summarizing the 800-year history of the rise of cats and madness, this chapter assesses the strength of the correlation between them. It does so by examining various epidemiolocal and genetic aspects of psychosis and asks how well these fit with *Toxoplasma gondii* as a possible etiological agent.

So what does English history tell us about cats and madness? In 1233 Pope Gregory issued a papal bull officially designating cats as being in league with Satan. Thereafter for almost 400 years, until the end of the Renaissance, cats were used to guard the grain but otherwise held in very low esteem. On Christian holidays they were often tortured or killed, and to keep a cat as a pet would brand the person as possibly being a witch. During these same years, occasional cases of madness were seen, caused by such things as brain infection, brain trauma, and nutritional deficiencies, as had been true for centuries. But until the end of the Renaissance, there were no suggestions that the incidence of madness was increasing.

The social status of cats began to improve in the seventeenth century as pet keeping became more common. Dogs and birds were the most common pets for most people but some aristocrats, clerics, poets, writers, and artists preferred cats. This trend was accentuated in the eighteenth century when leading intellectuals like Samuel Johnson and Horace Walpole kept cats, as did many of the leading poets, some of whom developed psychosis. For the first time, artists occasionally included cats in paintings of people, especially girls and women. The seventeenth century also saw a striking increase in interest in madness among the public. London's Elizabethan and Jacobian theater depicted madness in many plays. Visits to see the mad people in Bethlem Hospital became a staple for tourists to London; despite having less than 30 patients early in the century, it was widely visited and regarded as a human zoo. By 1676 it had become so overcrowded that a new hospital for 120 patients was built. Several other public psychiatric hospitals began opening, and private mad houses, as they were called, proliferated. All of this activity continued increasing in the eighteenth century. In 1742 it was estimated that 19,000 people

© E. Fuller Torrey 2022
E. F. Torrey, *Parasites, Pussycats and Psychosis*,
https://doi.org/10.1007/978-3-030-86811-6_6

were visiting Bethlem each year, and in 1770 the hospital was closed to visitors altogether because of the problems they were causing. In 1733 George Cheyne published *The English Malady* claiming that England had more mad people than any other country and that they were increasing rapidly. The book launched a spirited debate which would continue for almost 200 years.

In the nineteenth century, cats came into their own in England as valued pets. Queen Victoria kept cats along with many other pets, and cats continued to be popular among artists, poets and other writers, and among intellectuals in general. In 1871 the first national cat show was held in London, a measure of how far they had come since their association with Satan. The nineteenth century also witnessed a striking increase in the number of people diagnosed as insane and in public interest in this issue. In 1824 there had been just 8 public asylums in England; by 1890 there were 66, and by 1914 there were 97, each holding 10 times more patients than the original asylums. According to the official census counts of insane persons, there was a fivefold increase per population between 1829 and 1915. During the nineteenth century, the issue of rising insanity became a major concern of parliament and of the public in general.

Concern about rising insanity in the nineteenth century was not unique in England. In *The Invisible Plague*, we documented similar increases in Ireland, Canada, and the United States, and there are references to similar increases also having occurred in France and Germany. However, among these countries England has the best data on the history of cats as well as good records on the rise of insanity [1].

In examining the data in England for the seventeenth, eighteenth, and nineteenth centuries, there does indeed appear to be a correlation between the rise of cats and the rise of madness. Especially impressive is the increase in public interest, as measured by visits to Bethlem Hospital, suggesting that madness was a new phenomenon. Also impressive are the number of cases of psychosis that occurred among the poets and other writers who had pioneered the keeping of cats as pets.

However just because there is a correlation between the rise of cats and the rise of madness in England does not mean that there is necessarily any relationship, other than a statistical one, between the two. Correlation, in short, is not the same as causation. Two items might be correlated because they cause each other. For example, poverty and lack of education are correlated because they cause each other. Similarly, the sale of sunglasses and the sale of ice cream are correlated because they're both caused by the same thing—warm weather. There are also correlations that are purely accidental. In 2018 "Bloomberg News" published several classic examples of such correlations. For instance, from 2005 to 2011, the number of Facebook users was highly correlated with the Greek debt crisis. And from 1991 to 2009, the number of newborn girls named Ava was highly correlated with the US housing crisis [2].

How, then, can you determine when a correlation *does* indicate causation? Since the historic rise of cats is correlated with the rise of madness, how can one determine whether or not this is causal? The answer is that you must test for the plausibility of the relationship using other information. In this situation some examples of using other information includes the following. What do we know about the prevalence of psychosis among groups that do not keep cats as pets? What do we know about the prevalence of psychosis among groups that have very high rates of infection with *Toxoplasma gondii*? Can infection with *T. gondii* explain the epidemiological peculiarities of schizophrenia? For example, why are people who develop schizophrenia more likely to have been born in the winter or spring? Why are they twice as likely to have lived in an urban area, compared to a rural area, in childhood? Why are they more likely to live in a colder climate? In Europe, why is the prevalence of schizophrenia so high among some specific groups of immigrants? Schizophrenia and bipolar disorder are widely claimed to be primarily caused by genetics: can *Toxoplasma gondii* explain that? And, finally, since 40 million Americans are infected with *T. gondii* and we have approximately 140 million cats in the country, why isn't psychosis more common?

6.2   Fewer Cats, Less Psychosis?

In the 1960s Dr. Gordon Wallace studied the prevalence of cats and the prevalence of *Toxoplasma gondii* on remote islands in the Pacific Ocean. He established that on islands where cats had never existed, the parasite also did not exist. Similarly, on islands that had seen very few cats, the parasite appeared to be rare. This suggests that groups of people who have had little or no contact with cats should have a lower rate of psychosis insofar as *T. gondii* causes psychosis [3].

Are there any groups of people who have had minimal exposure to cats and on whom a psychosis prevalence survey has been carried out? The 800,000 people living in the highlands of Papua New Guinea in the 1970s met such criteria. They had had no contact with the outside world until after World War II when gold miners and missionaries began visiting. Since there were no indigenous felines in Papua New Guinea, these people had had no exposure to *T. gondii*.

In 1929 C. G. Seligman, a British anthropologist who had worked in Papua New Guinea, claimed that he had never seen a case of psychosis among individuals living in remote villages but had seen cases among individuals living along the coast among European traders and missionaries, many of whom had brought their cats with them. In the 1960s Dr. Carlton Gajdusek spent many months in the highlands of Papua New Guinea examining all neurologically impaired individuals in his study of kuru, for which he was later awarded a Nobel Prize. He said that in all of his studies there he had never seen a case of schizophrenia. Based on these reports, in 1973, I carried out a 2-month study of psychiatric patients in Papua New Guinea. With the assistance of the country's only psychiatrist, who had been there for 14 years, I reviewed all 1459 psychiatric case records covering the years 1970 to 1973. All cases of psychosis or probable psychosis were tabulated, with the total number being very low by international standards. I then ascertained the district of birth for all psychosis cases, comparing especially those who had been born in the highland districts, covering 800,000 people who had had possible contact with cats for only a few years, to those who had been born in the coastal districts, covering 1 million people who had had possible contact with cats for 50–70 years. For all cases of psychosis, the prevalence rate in individuals from the coastal districts was five times higher than the rate for individuals from the highland districts. For cases that met criteria for schizophrenia, the difference was tenfold. Thus in Papua New Guinea in 1973, a longer exposure to the elements of Western civilization, including possible exposure to cats, was a risk factor for developing psychosis [4].

Another group that has had minimal exposure to cats and on whom psychiatric surveys have been carried out is the Hutterites. They are an Anabaptist sect who migrated from Central Europe to the United States and Canada in 1874–1877. They reside communally in self-sufficient rural colonies living simple and austere lives. Traditionally they have kept no pets, considering it frivolous and unnecessary. When I visited two Hutterite colonies in 1994, a few older women living alone were beginning to keep small dogs as pets but not cats.

A detailed psychiatric survey had been carried out on the Hutterites in 1950–1953. At the time they numbered about 35,000. The prevalence rates for schizophrenia and bipolar disorder were very low by international standards, being 0.9 and 0.6 per 1000 population, respectively. A second detailed survey was carried out in 1992–1997 and reported rates of 1.2 per thousand for schizophrenia and 1.5 per thousand for affective psychosis. These rates are very low by international standards and suggest that having minimal exposure to cats results in a low prevalence of psychosis [5, 6].

6.3   More Toxoplasmosis, More Psychosis?

The fact that fewer cats are associated with less psychosis suggests that more toxoplasmosis might be associated with more psychosis. In fact, the seropositivity rate indicating past infection with *Toxoplasma gondii* varies widely from country to country. Studies in France and Ethiopia, for example, have reported rates of 80% or higher among some segments of the population, whereas other countries, such as China until recently, have reported rates of 10% or less. Most of these very high rates have been reported from countries where eating undercooked or raw meat is considered a delicacy among some people; France and Ethiopia both fall within this category. However neither France nor Ethiopia has an unusually elevated prevalence rate of psychosis according to studies done there. France has an average rate of psychosis by international standards, and in Ethiopia studies have reported below-average prevalence rates. Thus this would appear to be a strong argument that *Toxoplasma gondii* is not causally related to psychosis [7].

However, there is a possible explanation for this discrepancy. The form of the *Toxoplasma gondii* parasite that infects people when they ingest tissue cysts in undercooked meat is the bradyzoite form. This is quite different from the form of the parasite that infects people when they ingest or inhale oocysts in contaminated water, while playing in the sandbox, or gardening; that is the sporozoite form. Until recently it was not possible to tell whether an infected person had become infected from tissue cysts or oocysts, but newly developed assays now make this possible. Using these assays it is now known that most congenital forms of toxoplasmosis and most of the North American outbreaks have been caused by oocysts, not tissue cysts. As was mentioned in Chap. 2, studies in mice have shown that infections caused by oocysts are more severe than those caused by tissue cysts and there are suggestions that this is also true in humans. Thus it is possible, although not proven, that most cases of toxoplasma- associated psychosis are a consequence of oocyst infection. Insofar as this is true, one would not expect to see a correlation between *T. gondii* seropositivity rates and the prevalence of psychosis when the rates include both oocyst and tissue system infections [8].

6.4   Seasonality of Birth

One of the most clearly established aspects of schizophrenia and bipolar disorder is that there is a winter and spring excess of births for individuals who later develop these diseases. This was initially reported in 1929 in a study in Switzerland and 5 years later in the United States. More than 250 studies have since been done on this phenomena. The seasonal excess is a modest but highly significant 5–8% for the months of December through April in the northern hemisphere although in some countries for specific months it can be much higher. The seasonal excess is greater for schizophrenia than for bipolar disorder; is more pronounced for individuals born in urban areas; and more pronounced in countries farther away from the equator, for example, greater in Northern Europe than in Southern Europe. No adequate explanation has been offered for the seasonal phenomena. It is been shown that there is no seasonal predisposition to pregnancy among the parents, and the seasonal pattern is not more pronounced in families with a history of schizophrenia or bipolar disorder [9].

How might infection with *Toxoplasma gondii* explain this seasonal birth pattern? It is known that families keep cats indoors more in the winter than during the warmer weather. It is also thought by some researchers that when a cat becomes infected with *T. gondii* and is excreting millions of infective oocysts daily, the oocysts may become aerosolized when the cat feces dries out after about 24 hours. As such, the oocysts may be inhaled by individuals in the vicinity of the feces and cause clinical toxoplasmosis. As mentioned in Chap. 2, our appreciation of aerosolized oocysts as a threat has increased in recent years based on an outbreak at a riding stable in Atlanta and also by our ability to detect oocysts in an outdoor environment where cats have regularly defecated. Thus, just as pregnant women can become infected with toxoplasmosis by changing the cat litter so too might a newborn baby become infected by breathing in the oocysts, especially if the cat litter is in the same room with the newborn. The newborn might then develop toxoplasma brain cysts that could manifest as schizophrenia two decades later [10, 11].

6.5   Urban Living in Childhood

Another clearly established epidemiological aspect of schizophrenia is the risk of urban living in childhood. More than 20 studies have reported that children who lived in cities during childhood have twice the risk of later developing schizophrenia compared to those who lived in rural areas. The risk is also dose-dependent insofar as the more years the child lived in the city, the greater is the risk. Many explanations, including the stress of urban life, have been offered but none proven.

Since many cities have large numbers of feral cats and since cats prefer to deposit their feces in loose soil or sand, this may provide an explanation. Cities are covered with concrete and offer very few places for cats to defecate. Children's play areas on school grounds and in public parks would be attractive to cats. As will be detailed in the next chapter, studies have reported such areas as being highly infested with *T. gondii* oocysts. For example, a study of public sandboxes in Japan reported that there were estimated to be more than 1 million oocysts per square foot of sand. In rural areas, by contrast, cats have many more options regarding places to defecate so the concentration of oocysts would be less [12].

6.6   More Psychosis Where It's Colder

Still another established epidemiological aspect of psychosis is its association with colder climates. Multiple studies in Europe since the 1960s have reported that the incidence and prevalence of psychosis are higher in Northern Europe than it is in Southern Europe. This was most recently demonstrated by a large study of first episode psychosis at 16 sites in 5 European countries. The incidence of first episode nonaffective psychosis, most of whom have schizophrenia, was higher at the London site than at any other of the 16 sites and was 10 times higher than the incidence of the lowest site, which was Santiago in Spain. The incidence in other Northern European cities—Amsterdam and Paris—was also high, but it was not elevated in the Southern European cities of Madrid, Barcelona, Bologna, or Palermo. In general, the incidence rates at the sites in England, France, and the Netherlands were twice as high as those in Spain and Italy, thus confirming many older studies that have reported a higher incidence of schizophrenia in Northern Europe compared to Southern Europe. Although most such studies have been carried out in Europe, the same pattern was observed in the United States a century ago but has never been reexamined [13, 14].

One possible explanation for this striking north to south geographical gradient of psychosis is exposure to the *Toxoplasma gondii* oocysts. As noted above, in colder weather, cats are much more likely to be kept indoors and thus to defecate in cat litter. If the feces of an infected cat is allowed to dry out, the oocysts may become aerosolized, thereby exposing people living in the household to infection.

6.7   The Immigrant Issue

Among the most unusual findings in psychosis research in recent years have been reports of very high rates of psychosis among some, but not other, immigrant groups in European countries, especially in the Netherlands and England. Such studies have not been done in the United States. A striking example are studies of Caribbean immigrants to England. This unusual prevalence was first reported in 1965 and has been confirmed in many studies up to the present. A 1988 study, for example, reported the schizophrenia rate for Caribbean immigrants to be ten times higher than the rate for native-born English, and the rate for first-generation offspring of the Caribbean immigrants was even higher. Similarly, a recent study reported that "the incidence of all psychoses was over six times higher in African populations in the UK, compared with the British" [15–18].

How might these unusual findings be explained by infection with *Toxoplasma gondii*? It is known that the rate of exposure to *T. gondii* among people living in the Caribbean region is very high, as measured among pregnant women living there. A review of studies from ten English-speaking Caribbean countries reported that "a sizeable human population in the Caribbean becomes infected with *T. gondii* during childhood." However, the prevalence of schizophrenia is not unusually high there. Of special interest, however, is the fact that the predominant strains of the *T. gondii* parasite are different in the Caribbean than in England, and it is known that different strains can produce very different clinical outcomes. Whereas the type II strain is thought to be predominant in England as well as the United States, the type III and many atypical strains are predominant in the Caribbean. Since people can become infected with more than one strain, it may be a combination of strains that causes psychosis. Regarding the children of the Caribbean immigrants who are born in England and are also known to have a high incidence of psychosis, many of these children go back and forth between England and the Caribbean and often "live for some years with relatives at home," thus exposing them to *T. gondii* and other infectious agents in the Caribbean as well as in England [19–22].

6.8 Isn't Schizophrenia Genetic?

Textbooks of psychiatry now claim that schizophrenia and bipolar disorder are primarily genetic diseases. By this is meant that genes play a dominant role in the etiology, which for schizophrenia has been estimated by some geneticists to be 80% or greater. In fact schizophrenia is not primarily a genetic disease. It is of course a familial disease, meaning that it runs in families, but being familial is not the same as being genetic. Many traits can be familial but not genetic, such as speaking Spanish.

How do we know that schizophrenia is not primarily a genetic disease? One reason is that, despite the expenditure of literally hundreds of millions of dollars over two decades, no evidence has emerged to support schizophrenia as being primarily a genetic disease. As one critic described the research in 2016, "The current trend in psychiatric genetics is to use enormous samples to find genes of minuscule effect." In fact the strongest and most replicated schizophrenia genetic finding to date has been the findings in the MHC complex of chromosome 6 pointing to infectious, inflammatory, or immunologic factors as being of greatest importance [23, 24].

We also know that schizophrenia is not primarily a genetic disease because when you stop people who have schizophrenia from reproducing it has no effect on the subsequent incidence of the disease. For a full century, from the 1850s to the 1950s, we hospitalized most people with severe schizophrenia and did not allow them to reproduce. During that time in North America and Western Europe, the incidence of schizophrenia did not decrease but rather increased. In the United States between 1907 and 1940, more than 18,000 people with schizophrenia and bipolar disorder were sterilized, three quarters of them in the states of California, Kansas, and Virginia. However there is no evidence that the sterilizations had any effect on the future incidence of psychiatric disorders in those states or in the United States as a whole. The definitive test of the efficacy of eugenics for decreasing the incidence of schizophrenia was the horrific public policies of Nazi Germany. Between 1934 and 1945, it was estimated that 132,000 people with schizophrenia were sterilized and approximately an equal number were killed. This totaled at least three quarters of all individuals with schizophrenia in Germany prior to World War II. Postwar studies reported a low prevalence rate for schizophrenia, as expected, but a relatively high incidence of the disease. Thus eliminating reproduction by individuals with schizophrenia had no effect on the future incidence of the disease [25].

So how might *Toxoplasma gondii* run in families and thus be a familial disease but not be a genetic disease? As noted in Chap. 2, toxoplasmosis often runs in families, for example, from shared food such as undercooked lamb or raw goat's milk. Family outbreaks have also occurred from sharing an oocyst-contaminated water source. Extended families also often socialize together, thus exposing family members to a common risk factor. For example, the preschool children of an extended family in Alabama often played together in a yard with a toxoplasmosis-positive cat which had recently given birth to kittens. Seven of the nine preschool children were diagnosed with symptomatic toxoplasmosis. The common denominator of the children who became ill was a habit of putting sand or dirt in their mouth. A familial pattern of toxoplasmosis is also produced occasionally when an infected woman gives birth to two children who are congenitally infected; this may occur over a period of many years. There is also an intriguing pattern of familial toxoplasmosis which has been documented in mice. *Toxoplasma gondii* can be passed from generation to generation in mice, just as a gene would be, for as many as ten generations. Whether this also happens in humans is not known [26–28].

6.9   Why Isn't There More Psychosis?

Given the fact that 40 million Americans are infected with *Toxoplasma gondii* and that we have an estimated 140 million cats, wouldn't we expect psychosis to be more common if this parasite really does cause some cases of psychosis? In fact, we do not have very good information on the true prevalence of psychosis in the United States. The last reliable survey of this question was carried out by the National Institutes of Mental Health (NIMH) in the early 1980s and reported that 1.1% of adults or approximately 2.8 million people had schizophrenia at that time. A recent study, based on Medicaid and Medicare data, reported that 1.6% of the adult population, or approximately 3.8 million people, now have the symptoms of schizophrenia. This study did not include mentally ill individuals in jails and prisons of which, one study suggests, there may be another 200,000 individuals with schizophrenia.

Thus the total number of people with schizophrenia in the United States is probably about 4 million, and that number does not include individuals with psychosis associated with bipolar disorder or major depression. If *T. gondii* is responsible for causing even one quarter of these, that is a lot of psychosis [29].

Another consideration in regard to why there is not more psychosis is the fact that infectious diseases change over time. This is the theory of evolutionary epidemiology. According to this theory, "pathogen virulence and horizontal transmission is highest at the onset of an epidemic but decreases thereafter, as the epidemic depletes the pool of susceptible hosts." Thus the disease spreads most rapidly and is the most severe when it first becomes manifest. At some point in time, depending on the host characteristics and patterns of transmission, the incidence of the disease levels off. This has been demonstrated to occur in epidemics such as syphilis which was a much more severe disease when it was introduced in Europe in the early sixteenth century. Additional evidence that this is also true for schizophrenia is the fact that clinically it appears to have become a less severe disease in recent decades with fewer cases seen with catatonic or hebephrenic features and recovery occurring more frequently [30–32].

Returning to the original question, given the fact that there appears to be a correlation between the rise of cats and the rise of psychosis, is it likely that the correlation represents causation? By examining other aspects of psychosis, how well can they be explained by invoking *T. gondii*, a parasite carried by cats. In short, is the theory plausible? I believe the answer is yes, it is plausible.

References

1. Torrey EF, Miller J. The invisible plague: the rise and fall of mental illness from 1950 to the present. New Brunswick: Rutgers University Press, 343; 2002.
2. Chandrasekaran V. Correlation or causation? Bloomberg Businessweek, December 1, 2011.
3. Wallace GD. Serologic and epidemiologic observations on toxoplasmosis on three Pacific atolls. Am J Epidemiol. 1969;90(2):103–11. https://doi.org/10.1093/oxfordjournals.aje.a121054.
4. Torrey EF, et al. The epidemiology of schizophrenia in Papua New Guinea. Am J Psychiatry. 1974;131:567–73.
5. Nimgaonkar VL, et al. Low prevalence of psychoses among the Hutterites, an isolated religious community. Am J Psychiatry. 2000;157:1065–70. https://doi.org/10.1176/appi.ajp.157.7.
6. Torrey EF. Prevalence of psychosis among the Hutterites: a reanalysis of the 1950-53 study. Schizophr Res. 1995;16(2):167–70.
7. Saha S, et al. A systematic review of the prevalence of schizophrenia. PLoS Med. 2005;2(5):e141. https://doi.org/10.1371/journal.pmed.0020141.
8. Boyer K, et al. Unrecognized ingestion of *Toxoplasma gondii* oocysts leads to congenital toxoplasmosis and causes epidemics in North America. Clin Infect Dis Soc Am. 2011;53:1081–9.
9. Torrey EF, et al. Seasonality of births in schizophrenia and bipolar disorder: a review of the literature. Schizophr Res. 1997;28:1–38.
10. Lass A, et al. The first detection of *Toxoplasma gondii* DNA in environmental air samples using gelatine filters, real-time PCR and loop-mediated isothermal (LAMP) assays: qualitative and quantitative analysis. Parasitology. 2017;144(13):1791–801.
11. Teutsch SM, et al. Epidemic toxoplasmosis associated with infected cats. N Engl J Med. 1979;300(13):695–9.
12. Torrey EF, Yolken RH. The urban risk and migration risk factors for schizophrenia: are cats the answer? Schizophr Res. 2014;159:299–302.

13. Jongsme HE, et al. Treated incidence of psychotic disorders in the multinational EU-GEI study. JAMA Psychiat. 2018;75:36–46.
14. White WA. The geographical distribution of insanity in the United States. J Nerv Ment Dis. 1903;30:257–79.
15. Gordon EB. Mentally ill West Indian immigrants. Br J Psychiatry. 1965;111:877–87.
16. Harrison G, et al. A prospective study of severe mental disorder in Afro-Caribbean patients. Psychol Med. 1988;18:643–57.
17. Hutchinson G, Haason C. Migration and schizophrenia. Soc Psychiatry Psychiatr Epidemiol. 2004;39:350–7.
18. Kirkbride JB, et al. Incidence of schizophrenia and other psychoses in England, 1950–2009: a systematic review and meta-analysis. PLoS One. 2012;7:e31660. https://doi.org/10.1371/journal.pone.0031660.
19. Dubey JP, et al. Toxoplasmosis in the Caribbean Islands. Parasitol Res. 2016;115:1627–34.
20. Gilbert RE, et al. Prevalence of *Toxoplasma* IgG among pregnant women in West London according to country of birth and ethnic group. Br Med J. 1993;306:185–9.
21. Flatt A, Shetty N. Seroprevalence and risk factors for toxoplasmosis among antenatal women in London. Eur J Pub Health. 2012;23:648–52.
22. Moura L, et al. Seroprevalence of *Toxoplasma gondii* in cats from St. Kitts, West Indies. J Parasitol. 2007;93:952–3.
23. Leo J. The search for schizophrenia genes. Issues Sci Technol. 2016;32:68–72.
24. Corvin A, Morris DW. Genome-wide association studies: findings at the major histocompatibility complex locus in psychosis. Biol Psychiatry. 2014;75:276–83.
25. Torrey EF, Yolken RH. Psychiatric genocide: Nazi attempts to eradicate schizophrenia. Schizophr Bull. 2010;36:26–32.
26. Stagno S, et al. An outbreak of toxoplasmosis linked to cats. Pediatrics. 1980;65:706–12.
27. Beverley JKA. Congenital transmission of toxoplasmosis through successive generations of mice. Nature. 1959;183:1348–9.
28. Dubey JP. History of the discovery of the life cycle of *Toxoplasma gondii*. Int J Parasitol. 2009;39:877–82.
29. Mojtabai R. Estimating the prevalence of schizophrenia in the United States using the multiplier method. Lett Schizophr Res. 2021;240:48–9.
30. Berngruber TW, et al. Evolution of virulence in emerging epidemics. PLoS Pathog. 2013;9:e1003209.
31. Bolker BM, et al. Transient virulence of emerging pathogens. J R Soc Interface. 2010;7:811–22.
32. McGlashan TH. At issue: is natural selection rendering schizophrenia less severe? Schizophr Bull. 2006;32:428–9.

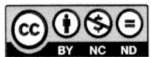

Sentinel Seals, Safe Cats, and Better Treatments

7

7.1   A Review

This chapter examines some additional implications of the *Toxoplasma gondii* problem. Especially impressive is evidence suggesting that this parasite is contaminating our land and waterways. The infection of marine mammals by this parasite is little known but disturbing. The chapter then proposes various solutions to the problem: specifically by better control of feral cats to decrease the distribution of *T. gondii* oocysts; by research, including the development of vaccines for cats; by improving the treatment of toxoplasmosis in humans; and by educating the public regarding these issues.

We began this story by establishing two preliminary facts. First, many human diseases are caused by infectious agents transmitted to us from animals, the Covid pandemic being the most recent example. Second, there is abundant evidence that infectious agents can cause psychosis. We then examined in detail *Toxoplasma gondii*, a protozoan parasite carried by cats. It is known to infect 40 million Americans, most of them apparently being asymptomatic. However, it has been clearly established that this parasite causes congenital problems of the central nervous system, estimated to be approximately 3800 cases per year in the United States, and is also a major cause of eye diseases, estimated to be approximately 4800 symptomatic cases per year. In addition, this parasite is a risk factor for causing cerebral toxoplasmosis in individuals who are immunosuppressed, including patients with HIV-AIDS, individuals receiving organ transplants, and cancer patients being treated with immunosuppressive drugs. Toxoplasmosis causes an estimated 71 deaths each year in the United States, mostly due to cerebral toxoplasmosis.

We then examined in detail the evidence linking *Toxoplasma gondii* to the cause of some cases of psychosis. Four facts are supportive of such a link. First, *Toxoplasma gondii* is known to cause psychotic symptoms. Next, among individuals with schizophrenia, those who are infected with this parasite have been shown to have more severe symptoms. Third, many studies have shown that individuals with psychosis, compared to controls, are significantly more likely to have antibodies against

© E. Fuller Torrey 2022
E. F. Torrey, *Parasites, Pussycats and Psychosis*,
https://doi.org/10.1007/978-3-030-86811-6_7

this parasite, indicating a past infection. Finally, some but not all studies have reported that adults with psychosis, compared to controls, were significantly more likely as children to have lived in a house with cats.

To further explore a possible link between *Toxoplasma gondii* and psychosis, we next looked at the unusual 800-year history of cats which transitioned from being perceived as agents of Satan to becoming cherished pets. We found that there appears to be a correlation between the historic rise of cats as pets and the increasing incidence of psychosis. Finally, we examined several epidemiological aspects of schizophrenia, such as the fact that it is more common in cold climates, to ascertain whether these aspects can be explained by infection with *Toxoplasma gondii*. Overall, the evidence linking this parasite to the cause of some case of psychosis is strong. One estimate of the number of cases of psychosis that might be linked to *Toxoplasma gondii* suggested about 20%, or 15,000 new cases of psychosis each year in the United States.

In addition to examining the possible link between *Toxoplasma gondii* and psychosis, we also briefly reviewed studies that have attempted to link this parasite to other diseases and conditions. The strongest evidence for a *T. gondii* link from studies done to date is for some cases of brain cancer, epilepsy, and rheumatoid arthritis. In addition, a small number of motor vehicle accidents may be linked to *T. gondii* based on the fact that the parasite slows human reaction times.

In summary, the importance of this relatively unknown parasite has been greatly underestimated, especially given the fact that it is known to infect approximately 40 million Americans. The next step is to ascertain the magnitude of the toxoplasmosis problem.

7.2   What Is the Magnitude of the Problem?

Since cats are the definitive host for *T. gondii*, solutions to the problems caused by this parasite will inevitably involve them. As noted in Chap. 1, the United States is thought to have approximately 90 million owned cats and 50 million feral cats for a total of 140 million. Studies have reported that the fecal production of a cat is approximately 40 grams per day. Thus the total daily fecal production for all the cats in the United States would be approximately 5.6 billion grams. Converted into pounds this would be 12,334,800 million pounds or 6167 tons. To visualize this, imagine a train with 62 standard boxcars, each of which carries 100 tons of freight. Then imagine the freight train being two thirds of a mile in length; this is what would be required to carry 1 days' fecal output for all the cats in the United States [1, 2].

Studies have shown that at any given time approximately 1% of all cats are excreting oocysts. One percent of 5.6 billion grams is 56 million grams of oocyst-infected cat feces which would be produced each day in the United States. Each gram of infected cat feces may contain between 1 million and 13 million oocysts; assuming a mean of 6 million oocysts per gram for the 56 million grams of infected cat feces would produce a total of 336 trillion (336,000,000,000) *T. gondii* oocysts each day. Although it is not known how many oocysts are needed to infect a human, studies have been done in pigs which weigh about the same as humans, and it only took one oocyst to infect them [3, 4].

One of the most striking aspects of *T. gondii* oocysts is their viability. They are remarkably hearty, especially if they are deposited in shady, moist, and temperate conditions. In Texas, under outdoor shaded conditions with a mean air temperature of 19.5 °C, oocysts remained viable during a 13-month experiment. In Kansas, oocysts were buried in loose soil and remained viable for 18 months. Oocysts maintained experimentally at 4 °C in seawater or freshwater remained viable for 24 and 54 months, respectively. Oocysts also survived for over a year in vials of 2% sulfuric acid at 4 °C. Because almost all of these studies were terminated while at least some of the oocysts were still viable, we really do not yet know the outer limit of viability for *T. gondii* oocysts deposited under various environmental conditions. What we do know is that many oocysts are infective for a long time [5–9].

7.3 Oocyst Contamination of Soil and Water

Given the fact that cats in the United States produce 336 trillion *T. gondii* oocysts each day and that some of these oocysts may survive for 2 years or longer, it is important to consider the fate of these oocysts. In urban and suburban areas, the majority would be deposited in loose soil in gardens or in public or private children's play areas or sandboxes. In rural areas the oocysts might be deposited in feed piles in the barn or in loose soil in the field, there to be ingested by grazing animals such as cows and sheep. In recent years many studies have been carried out to assess the degree of contamination of soil and water by the oocysts. Because the various studies used different methods of sampling and measurements of *T. gondii*'s presence, the results of the studies cannot be usefully compared with each other.

In California in Santa Cruz and Santa Clara Counties, six public parks and a community garden were sampled for *T. gondii* oocysts during the spring, summer, and fall seasons. Feral cat colonies were known to frequent all seven sites which were heavily used for public recreation. Three of the seven sites had positive samples for *T. gondii,* all in the fall season. At the Santa Cruz State Park, 20 of 27 samples were positive. Another study in California was carried out in three communities in the Morro Bay region. Among 12,244 households, researchers identified 7284 owned cats and an additional 2046 feral cats. Based on the information regarding cat defecation and cat litter disposition in these communities, the researchers calculated that the oocyst burden for the land area of residential housing ranged between 9 and 434 oocysts per square foot of land area [10–12].

Studies from several other countries clearly confirm that soil contamination by *T. gondii* oocysts is now worldwide. A study similar to the Morro Bay study was carried out in three communities in rural France and reported a similar oocyst burden of between 3 and 335 oocysts per square foot. In Brazil, *T. gondii* oocysts were isolated from ten soil samples taken from the playgrounds of 31 elementary schools; the authors suggested that these results indicated a wide distribution of *T. gondii* oocysts around elementary schools in the region. In a village in Panama, it was estimated that the oocyst burden in soil near houses where cats were regularly fed varied from 18 to 72 per square foot. In Poland, *T. gondii* oocysts were isolated from 18 of 101 soil samples taken from places thought to be favored by cats for defecation: sandboxes, playgrounds, parks, gardens, and areas around rubbish dumps. In Iran *T. gondii* DNA was identified in 18 of 200 soil samples taken from public parks, playgrounds, sand pits, and around rubbish dumps. In Pakistan *T. gondii* DNA was found in 42 of 250 soil samples taken from parks, playgrounds, and sandpits where children play. In China *T. gondii* was found in 58 of 252 soil samples taken from 6 public parks in Wuhan. Finally, a recent study from 6 provinces in China reported the results of soil sampling from 420 sites at schools, parks, farms, and coastal beaches. Out of the 420 sites, 136 (32%) were positive for *T. gondii* DNA. The evidence of high soil contamination in the Chinese samples is especially concerning since keeping pet cats under Chairman Mao was discouraged and has only become common in the last two decades. A recent review of 22 such studies concluded: "The results are a cause for concern because various areas studied across the world are rather highly contaminated with toxoplasma oocysts" [13–22].

The loose sand in children's sandboxes/sandpits are especially attractive to cats as places to defecate. A study in Japan quantified the frequency of cat defecations in three public sandboxes by using night lights and a camcorder. Over almost 5 months, they recorded 961 cat defecations in the sandboxes. Assuming that 1% of the cats were shedding oocysts when they defecated and that the oocysts remained viable for at least 18 months, it is possible that the oocyst contamination in such a sandbox could reach over 1 million oocysts per square foot. Given the frequency with which young children put their fingers in their mouth, the chances of becoming infected with toxoplasmosis while playing in such a sandbox would be very high [23, 24].

However, it is not only soil samples that are being contaminated by *T. gondii* oocysts. Streams, rivers, and even the ocean are becoming contaminated to a remarkable degree. This occurs when cat feces are carried by rainwater into waterways and also when cat litter is flushed down the toilet. Increasingly, this is resulting in oocyst contamination of drinking water. In 1995, for example, a drinking water reservoir on Vancouver Island became contaminated with *T. gondii* oocysts resulting in at least 2984 human infections of which 100 had symptomatic toxoplasmosis. Contamination of drinking water reservoirs by *T. gondii* has also led to several outbreaks of toxoplasmosis in Brazil, including 1 involving 290 cases and another involving 155 cases [25, 26].

The consequences of the runoff of infected cat feces into the ocean have become abundantly clear. Between 1998 and 2004 along the California coast, 52% of the dead and 38% of the live sea otters tested were infected with *T. gondii*. One of the consequences of such infections is that sea otters infected with *T. gondii* have been shown to be almost four times more likely to be attacked by sharks compared to sea otters not infected. It is thought that the *T. gondii* in the cat feces are taken up by mussels and other shellfish which are then eaten by the sea mammals. And it is not just sea otters. Between 2004 and 2009, 161 mostly stranded sea mammals on the coast of Oregon, Washington, and southern British Columbia were examined. They included 95 seals, 37 porpoises, 19 sea lions, 5 sea otters, 4 whales, and 1 dolphin. Ninety-four of the 161, or 58%, were found to be infected with *T. gondii*. On the other side of the North American continent between 2009 and 2012 in the estuary of the St. Lawrence River, 34 beached beluga whales were tested. Fifteen of the 34, or 44%, were found to be infected with *T. gondii*. It was hypothesized that the source of the infection was cat feces from the estimated 2 million cats in Quebec, especially from the downriver urban Montreal area. *T. gondii* was also said to be responsible for the death of 406 seals in 2012 off the coast of Nova Scotia [27–31].

A summary of the studies published in 2020 makes abundantly clear how extensively toxoplasmosis has infected marine mammals. Based on antibody studies, at least nine marine mammal species have been proven to be infected with *T. gondii*: seals, sea otters, dolphins, porpoises, manatees, sea lions, whales, walruses, and dugong. Based on autopsy reports, toxoplasmosis has been proven to be the definitive or a contributory cause of death in some mammals in all of these species except the last two. For example, in southern sea otters, an endangered species, *T. gondii* was reported to be the primary cause of death for 17% and a contributory factor for an additional 12% based on sea otter deaths examined histologically between 1998 and 2001. And the effect is worldwide. Infected dolphins, for example, have been found off the coasts of the United States, Canada, Mexico, England, Spain, Italy, Russia, and the Philippines [32].

The contamination of the ocean by *T. gondii* from cat feces off the coasts of highly populated areas is alarming enough, but the situation is even worse. In 2014 it was announced that a beluga whale taken by Inuit hunters in the Beaufort Sea north of Alaska had tested positive for *T. gondii*. In recent decades cats have become popular pets in Eskimo communities. And in Antarctica 52% of Weddell seals and 23% of elephant seals have been found to be infected with *T. gondii*. Since the seals migrate, it is unknown where they became infected; one possibility is Macquarie Island which lies halfway between Antarctica and New Zealand. For many years the island was overrun with feral cats, the consequences of their introduction in the early nineteenth century by seal harvesters. As one recent paper concluded, "It is evident from the review that contamination of marine aquatic life with *T. gondii* is widespread and we are surrounded by a sea of toxoplasma" [33–35].

7.4 Solutions to the Problem

Given what we know and, more important, what we don't know about toxoplasmosis, it does not seem wise to be contaminating our land and water with infective oocysts. As a veterinary problem, we know that all warm-blooded animals can be infected and that it is a major cause of fetal loss in sheep and goats. As a human problem, we know that 40 million Americans are infected and that the infective oocysts are a significant cause of congenital brain problems, eye disease, and encephalitis for individuals who are immunocompromised due to HIV-AIDS, organ transplantation, or cancer treatment. Additional evidence suggests that toxoplasma may well play a role in causing some cases of psychosis as well as possibly causing some cases of brain cancer, epilepsy, rheumatoid arthritis, and even a few motor vehicle accidents. *Toxoplasma gondii* is clearly affecting animals and humans in ways we are just beginning to understand, and common sense would suggest we should not be contaminating our environment with the infective oocysts. Perhaps we should use the seals and other sea mammals that are dying on our beaches, many infected with toxoplasmosis, as sentinels. As a past generation used a canary in the coal mine as a sentinel, this generation might use a dead seal on a beach.

Solutions to the toxoplasmosis problem involve *four priority actions*.

7.4.1 Decrease the Distribution of Infective *T. gondii* Oocysts

The first is to decrease the distribution of the infective *T. gondii* oocysts in the environment. Since this distribution is being done by infected cats, the decrease can only be accomplished by decreasing the number of infected cats. Owned cats that are exclusively indoor cats are not a problem. They could theoretically become infected with *T. gondii* indoors if they caught a mouse that was infected, but the likelihood of this happening is low. Owned cats that go outdoors are a problem insofar as a significant percentage of them will become infected, most often at the time when they are starting to hunt. For such cats it is essential that the cat litter be cleaned each day, before the feces has dried and the oocysts have become aerosolized, and disposed of in the garbage, not flushed down the toilet. The ultimate solution to having a safe indoor and outdoor cat is the development of an effective vaccine, as will be described below.

The major source of the distribution of *T. gondii* oocysts in the environment are unowned and feral cats. Some of these cats were owned by people at one time but ran away or were left behind when the people moved, but the majority of them were never owned. As previously noted they are estimated to number between 30 and 80 million in the United States. Feral cats are not only responsible for a disproportionate share of the *T. gondii* oocysts being widely distributed on the land and in the water, they are also responsible for a disproportionate share of feline killings of birds and small mammals such as mice, squirrels, and rabbits. In the United States, it has been estimated that cats kill between 1 and 4 billion birds and between 6 and 22 billion small mammals each year; of this total, two thirds have been attributed to feral cats. Cats are highly effective predators; for example, a single feral cat was shown to have killed 46 out of 52 chickens on 1 farm over 4 nights. In Australia, which is estimated to have 2.7 million owned cats and at least 2 million feral cats, studies have shown that each year the feral cats kill 400 million birds and more than half a billion native mammals. According to one summary of the problem, "Overall, cats have played a major role in the extinction of 27 Australian species since European settlement and are currently threatening the existence of scores more" [36, 37].

Attempts to control the feral cat problem using humane methods have been unsuccessful. Most widely used have been programs that trap, neuter, and return feral cats to the wild. Multiple careful studies of these "TNR" programs, as they are known, have demonstrated that they don't work. Despite the dedicated work of volunteers who staff these programs, feral cats are difficult to trap, and neutering is expensive. Cats also reproduce faster than TNR programs can keep up with. The average female cat can become pregnant at 6 months of age, have a pregnancy lasting 9 weeks, and give birth to 3–6 kittens. She can then become pregnant again as soon as 4 weeks after giving birth. It is not uncommon for a female cat to have three litters a year. Indoor cats live on average for 12 to 18 years, feral cats much shorter depending on the conditions. Given its fertility, it is quite possible for a single female cat to have more than 1000 descendants by the time she dies [38].

The only effective means that has been found to date for controlling the cat population has been the killing of unwanted and feral cats. In the United States, approximately 1 million cats are euthanized each year in animal shelters overrun by such cats. A realistic solution to the feral cat problem would involve a significant increase in the number of cats euthanized. Given the passionate feelings of animal lovers in general, and cat lovers in particular, this will be difficult to do.

7.4.2 Research

A second priority for solving the toxoplasmosis problem is research. As noted above, the development of a vaccine against *T. gondii* is essential. Ideally it should be a vaccine that can be given to kittens to prevent them from ever becoming infected. Such cats would be regarded as safe pets for both children and adults, even if the cats could go outside. Farmers who keep cats in the barn would also vaccinate their kittens so that the animal feed would not become contaminated by infective oocysts. Developing a vaccine for kittens could be done using a live, attenuated strain of the parasite. Such a vaccine has been developed for use in sheep for which toxoplasmosis is a major cause of abortion; it is available in United Kingdom and some other countries but not in the United States or Canada. The development of a vaccine for kittens would not be easy because of the many strains of *T. gondii* and because the parasite is much more complex than a virus. However the recent success of vaccine development against the SARS-CoV-2 virus demonstrated what can be done when such a task is prioritized [39–41].

Unfortunately, in April 2019, animal rights activists made vaccine development more difficult. They lobbied members of congress and convinced them to introduce legislation, called the KITTEN Act, to close the toxoplasmosis research laboratory under the US Department of Agriculture because it was using cats as research subjects. This laboratory, which had been doing research on toxoplasmosis since 1982, was the single most important American research laboratory on this disease and its closure is a major setback for such research [42].

Much research needs to be done on human toxoplasmosis. If it can be proven to be causing even 20% of cases of new onset psychosis, that would be a huge step forward for psychiatric research since such cases could theoretically be prevented.

Also needed is additional research on whether *T. gondii* infection has an effect on personality characteristics, as some studies have reported, for individuals who are otherwise asymptomatic. For example, are there groups of Americans who have pronounced personality traits such as suspiciousness, impulsivity, or aggressiveness not because this is their normal personality but rather because they are infected with *T. gondii*? Related questions that need clarification include possible different effects of infection by a tissue cyst or an oocyst, the different effects of the many strains of the parasite, and the importance of the timing of the initial infection. For example, does an infection in children lead to a different outcome than an infection in adults? Research is also needed on the oocysts themselves. For example, how important is transmission by aerosolized oocysts in causing human disease? How important are the host genetics in determining the outcome of *T. gondii* infections? And how important are coinfections with other infectious agents in determining the outcome? In addition to research on psychosis, research is also needed on the other conditions linked by antibody studies to *T. gondii*—specifically brain cancer, epilepsy, rheumatoid arthritis, and motor vehicle accidents.

7.4.3   Better Treatments

The third priority action needed to solve the toxoplasmosis problem is the development of better treatments. The standard treatment for infections with *T. gondii* is pyrimethamine, trade name Daraprim, a drug also used to treat malaria. For treating toxoplasmosis pyrimethamine is usually used in combination with sulfadiazine or another sulfonamide antibiotic. For treating infections anywhere except the brain, this combination is moderately effective for most cases but there are significant side effects. For those who cannot tolerate the drug and those who are allergic to sulfa, a variety of other antiparasitic and antibiotic drugs have been tried but none have been better than pyrimethamine. However when *T. gondii* infects the brain, it is a different story. The blood-brain barrier blocks many drugs from getting into the brain. Furthermore, in the brain, *T. gondii* forms tissue cysts which are metabolically relatively inactive and therefore do not respond well to treatment by many drugs. The bottom line is that we currently have no effective treatment for infections by *T. gondii* in the brain [43].

Still another problem is the availability of pyrimethamine. This drug was first approved for use in the United States in 1953. For many years it was marketed by GlaxoSmithKline and sold for $1.00 a pill. In 2010 Glaxo sold the American marketing rights of Daraprim to CorePharma, which in 2014 sold them to Impax Laboratories, by which time the price of Daraprim had risen to $13.50 a pill. In 2015 Impax sold the rights to Turing Pharmaceuticals, a startup company run by a former hedge fund manager. Turing immediately raised the price of Daraprim to $750 a pill, thereby landing itself on the front page of the *New York Times* as another example of a pharmaceutical company legally but outrageously price gouging. Since that time the availability of pyrimethamine in the United States has been less predictable and, for many, unaffordable [44].

Given the need for better drugs to treat psychosis, a few attempts have been made to treat patients with schizophrenia using drugs thought to be effective against *T. gondii*. Between 2009 and 2014, four such randomly controlled trials were reported. Two trials used antibiotics—azithromycin and trimethoprim—and the other two trials used antiparasitic drugs, artemisinin and artemether. None of the four trials reported significant improvement in the symptoms of individuals with schizophrenia. This was not surprising given the fact that none of the four drugs have good penetration into the brain. In addition, three of the four trials used patients who had been sick for many years. To be effective it is quite possible that an anti-toxoplasma drug would have to be given in the earlier stages of the illness [45].

Thus there are many reasons to develop better drugs for the treatment of infections by *T. gondii*. But developing better drugs is expensive and generally only done by the pharmaceutical industry or government. The pharmaceutical industry apparently views the problems caused by human toxoplasmosis as being too small to be economically attractive. In the United States, the National Institutes of Health (NIH) unfortunately also regards human toxoplasmosis as being a low priority. This is demonstrated by the Research, Condition, and Disease Categorization (RCDC) database, a list of 292 diseases and conditions for which NIH provides annual data on how much is being spent for research. Among the 292 diseases and conditions, toxoplasmosis does not even make the list. If better drugs are to be developed for the treatment of toxoplasmosis, they are more likely to be developed in Europe or Asia than in the United States.

One place in which to look for better treatments for toxoplasmosis is the development of better antipsychotics. The chemical structure of many effective antiparasitic drugs is very similar to the structure of antipsychotic drugs. As early as 1891, it was reported that the phenothiazine dye, methylene blue, was effective in suppressing the parasite that causes malaria. Sixty years later the first effective antipsychotic, chlorpromazine, was developed; it is also a phenothiazine. Based on this history, we tested 12 antipsychotic and mood stabilizer drugs to ascertain their effectiveness in inhibiting *T. gondii* in cell culture. All of the 12 drugs except lithium demonstrated some ability to inhibit *T. gondii*, and two of them—the antipsychotic haloperidol and the mood stabilizer valproate—were even more effective than the antibiotic trimethoprim which is used to treat toxoplasmosis and was used in the study as the comparator drug. Thus it is possible that some of the effectiveness of antipsychotic drugs used to treat psychosis comes from the ability to suppress *T. gondii* or other infectious agents. And it is also possible that the ultimate solution to the toxoplasmosis treatment problem will come from the development of better antipsychotics [46].

Given the complexity of the *T. gondii* organism and its many strains, it will not be easy to develop better treatments for this parasite, but it can be done. One approach is to chemically modify compounds which are already known to possess some antiprotozoal activity. Recent published examples of this approach include studies on endochin-like quinolones [47]; 4-arylquinoline-2-carboxylate derivatives [48]; and a thiazole derivative of artemisinin [49]. Another approach is to screen large numbers of existing drugs and other chemical compounds to ascertain which ones have the best ability to inhibit *T. gondii* in cell culture. This approach has also identified large numbers of potentially useful anti-toxoplasma compounds [50–52].

7.4.4 Education

A fourth priority action for solving the toxoplasmosis problem is education. *Toxoplasma gondii* is virtually unknown in the United States except by women who have been pregnant and educated by their obstetricians. Thus most people have no knowledge of the role of cats and oocysts in spreading the disease. For example, animal lovers living in coastal communities will often make great efforts to save the lives of beached seals or other marine mammals, some of which were beached because they were infected with *T. gondii*. Some of these people will then go home and let their cat out. The cat's feces may then be washed by rainwater into a nearby stream that empties into the bay, thereby infecting more seals that may also beach themselves.

Toxoplasmosis-related problems could be significantly reduced in United States if the public was aware of the following facts.

- Cats that have been kept indoors from birth are safe pets for both children and adults.
- Cats that are allowed to go outside are likely to become infected with *T. gondii*, most often when they're starting to learn to hunt. In most cases the infected cat will have no symptoms, so the owner will have no way of knowing that the cat is infected.
- Feces from a cat litter box should be removed each day, put in a bag, and put in the garbage. It should never be flushed down the toilet.
- Pregnant women and people who are immunocompromised should never clean the cat litter box.
- Sandboxes and loose soil in children's play areas should always be covered when not in use.
- Gloves should be worn when gardening.
- Meat and seafood should be thoroughly cooked.
- Fruits that cannot be peeled and vegetables should be thoroughly washed before eating.
- Finally, treat cats as cats. Real cats are not like Garfield or Rum Tum Tugger, and they are not small humans with fur. They are a different animal species from humans, and it is possible to show affection for them without kissing them on the face. As noted in Chap. 1, cats are known to carry at least 273 infectious agents, 151 of which are known to be shared with humans. That's a heavy burden for a small animal and perhaps that is what made Grumpy Cat grumpy.

Given what we now know about toxoplasmosis, isn't it time to implement these actions?

References

1. Dabritz HA, Conrad PA. Cats and toxoplasmosis: implications for public health. Zoonoses Public Health. 2010;57:34–52.
2. Standard boxcars are 55.5 feet in length and there are 2 feet between the boxcars, thus making a train 3,565 feet or .68 miles in length.
3. Dubey JP. Toxoplasmosis of animals and humans. New York: CRC Press; 2010. p. 36, 38.
4. Dubey JP, et al. Infectivity of low numbers of *Toxoplasma gondii* oocysts to pigs. J Parasitol. 1996;82:438–43.
5. Yilmaz SM, Hopkins SH. Effects of different conditions on duration of infectivity on *Toxoplasma gondii* oocysts. J Parasitol. 1972;58:938–9.
6. Frenkel JK, et al. Soil survival of Toxoplasma oocysts in Kansas and Costa Rica. Am J Trop Med Hyg. 1975;24:439–43.
7. Dubey JP. *Toxoplasma gondii* oocyst survival under defined temperatures. J Parasitol. 1998;84:862–5.
8. Lindsey DS, Dubey JP. Long-term survival of *Toxoplasma gondii* sporulated oocysts in seawater. J Parasitol. 2009;95:1019–20.
9. Frenkel JK, Dubey JP. Toxoplasma and its prevention in cats and men. J Infect Dis. 1972;126:664–73.
10. de Wit LA, et al. Seasonal and spatial variation in *Toxoplasma gondii* contamination in soil in urban public spaces in California, United States. Zoonoses Public Health. 2020;67(1):70–8. https://doi.org/10.1111/zph.12656.
11. Dabritz HA, et al. Outdoor fecal deposition by free-roaming cats and attitudes of cat owners and nonowners toward stray pets, wildlife, and water pollution. J Am Vet Med Assoc. 2006;229(1):74–81. https://doi.org/10.2460/javma.229.1.74.
12. Dabritz HA, et al. Detection of *Toxoplasma gondii*-like oocysts in cat feces and estimates of the environmental oocyst burden. J Am Vet Med Assoc. 2007;231(11):1676–84. https://doi.org/10.2460/javma.231.11.1676.
13. Afonso E, et al. Local meteorological conditions, dynamics of seroconversion to *Toxoplasma gondii* in cats (*Felis catus*) and oocyst burden in rural environment. Epidemiol Infect. 2010;138:1105–13.
14. dos Santos TR, et al. Detection of *Toxoplasma gondii* oocysts in environmental samples from public schools. Vet Parasitol. 2010;171:53–7.
15. Sousa OE, et al. Toxoplasmosis in Panama: A 10 year study. Am J Trop Med Hyg. 1988;38:315–22.
16. Pacheco-Ortega GA, et al. Screening of zoonotic parasites in playground sandboxes of public parks from subtropical Mexico. J Parasitol Res. 2019;2019:7409076. https://doi.org/10.1155/2019/7409076.
17. Lass A, et al. Detection of *Toxoplasma gondii* oocysts in environmental soil sample using molecular methods. Eur J Clin Microbiol Infect Dis. 2009;28:599–605.
18. Du F, et al. Survey on the contamination of *Toxoplasma gondii* oocysts in the soil of public parks in Wuhan, China. Vet Parasitol. 2012;184:141–6.
19. Saki J, et al. Detection and genotyping of *Toxoplasma gondii* isolated from soil in Ahvaz, Southwest of Iran. J Parasitol Dis. 2017;41:202–5.
20. Ajmal A, et al. Detection of *Toxoplasma gondii* in environmental matrices (water, soil forests and vegetables). Afr J Microbiol Res. 2013;7:1505–11.
21. Cong W, et al. Prevalence, risk factors and genotype distribution of *Toxoplasma gondii* DNA in soil in China. Ecotoxicol Environ Saf. 2020;189:109999. https://doi.org/10.1016/j.ecoenv.2019.109999.
22. Maleki B, et al. Toxoplasma oocysts in the soil of public places worldwide: a systematic review and metanalysis. Trans R Soc Trop Med Hyg. 2021;115:471–81.
23. Uga S, et al. Defecation habits of cats and dogs and contamination by *Toxocara* eggs in public park sandpits. Am J Trop Med Hyg. 1996;54:122–6.

24. Torrey EF, Yolken RH. *Toxoplasma* oocysts as a public health problem. Trends Parasitol. 2013;29:380–4.
25. Bowie WR, et al. Outbreak of toxoplasmosis associated with municipal drinking water. The BC Toxoplasma investigation team. Lancet (London, England). 1997;350(9072):173–7. https://doi.org/10.1016/s0140-6736(96)11105-3.
26. Shapiro K, et al. Environmental transmission of *Toxoplasma gondii*: oocysts in water, soil and food. Food and Waterborne Parasitol. 2019;15:e00049. https://doi.org/10.1016/j.fawpar.2019.e00049.
27. Miller MA, et al. An unusual genotype of *Toxoplasma gondii* is common in California sea otters (Enhydra lutris nereis) and is a cause of mortality. Int J Parasitol. 2004;34(3):275–84. https://doi.org/10.1016/j.ijpara.2003.12.008.
28. Gibson AK, et al. Polyparasitism is associated with increased disease severity in *Toxoplasma gondii*-infected marine sentinel species. PLoS Negl Trop Dis. 2011;5:e1142. https://doi.org/10.1371/journal.pntd.0001142.
29. Dabritz HA, et al. Outdoor fecal deposition by free-roaming cats and attitudes of cat owners and nonowners toward stray pets, wildlife, and water pollution. J Am Vet Med Assoc. 2006;229:74–80.
30. Jessup DA, et al. Sea otters in a dirty ocean. J Am Vet Med Assoc. 2007;231:1648–52.
31. Iqbal A, et al. *Toxoplasma gondii* infection in stranded St. Lawrence Estuary beluga *Delphinapterus leucas* in Quebec, Canada. Dis Aquat Org. 2018;130:165–75.
32. Dubey JP, et al. Recent epidemiologic and clinical importance of *Toxoplasma gondii* infections in marine mammals: 2009–2020. Vet Parasitol. 2020;288:109296. https://doi.org/10.1016/j.vetpar.2020.109296.
33. Cat Parasite Found in Western Arctic Belugas. CBC News. February 17, 2014. https://www.cbc.ca/news/technology/cat-parasite-found-in-western-arctic-belugas-1.2536234.
34. Petersen DR, et al. Prevalence of activity to Toxoplasma among Alaska natives: relation to exposure to the felidae. J Infect Dis. 1974;130:557–63.
35. Jensen S-K, et al. Prevalence of *Toxoplasma gondii* antibodies in pinnipeds from Antarctica. Vet Rec. 2012;171:249. https://doi.org/10.1136/vr.100848.
36. Losos JB. Deadly cats down under: science meets the great cat debate. Science. 2019;375:328–9. https://doi.org/10.1126/science.aay2196.
37. Strycker N. To save birds should we kill off cats. National Geographic. 2019. Vol. 236. https://www.nationalgeographic.com/animals/2019/09/essay-to-save-birds-should-we-kill-off-cats/.
38. Read JL. Among the pigeons: why our cats belong indoors. Mile End: Wakefield Press; 2019. p. 111–30.
39. Li Y, Zhou H. Moving toward improved vaccines for *Toxoplasma gondii*. Expert Opin Biol Ther. 2018;18:273–80.
40. Singh T, et al. Vaccines for perinatal and congenital infections-how close are we? Front Pediatr. 2020;8:569. https://doi.org/10.3389/fped.2020.
41. Chu K-B, Quan F-S. Advances in *Toxoplasma gondii* vaccines: current strategies and challenges for vaccine development. Vaccine. 2021;9:413. https://doi.org/10.3390/vaccines9050413.
42. Wadman M. Closure of U.S. Toxoplasma lab draws ire. Science. 2019;364:109.
43. Neville AJ, et al. Clinically available medicines demonstrating anti-Toxoplasma activity. Antimicrob Agents Chemother. 2015;59:7161–9.
44. Pollack A. Once a neglected treatment, now an expensive specialty drug. The New York Times, September 21, 2015.
45. Chorlton SD. *Toxoplasma gondii* and schizophrenia: a review of published RCTs. Parasitol Res. 2017;116:1793–9.
46. Jones-Brando L, Torrey EF, Yolken R. Drugs used in the treatment of schizophrenia and bipolar disorder inhibit the replication of *Toxoplasma gondii*. Schizophr Res. 2003;62:237–44.
47. Doggett SJ, et al. Endochin-like quinolones are highly efficacious against acute and latent experimental toxoplasmosis. Proc Natl Acad Sci. 2012;109:15936–41.
48. McNulty J, et al. Synthesis and anti-toxoplasmosis activity of 4-arylquinoline-2-carboxylate derivatives. Org Biomol Chem. 2014;12(2):255–60.

49. Schultz TL, et al. A thiazole derivative of artemisinin moderately reduces *Toxoplasma gondii* cyst burden in infected mice. J Parasitol. 2014;100:516–21.
50. Hencken CP, et al. Thiazole, oxadiazole, and carboxamide derivatives of artemisinin are highly selective and potent inhibitors of *Toxoplasma gondii*. J Med Chem. 2010;53:3594–601.
51. Adeyemi OS, et al. Screening of chemical compound libraries identified new anti-*Toxoplasma gondii* agents. Parasitol Res. 2018;117:355–63.
52. Murata Y, et al. Identification of compounds that suppress *Toxoplasma gondii* tachyzoites and bradyzoites. PloS One. 2017. https://doi.org/10.1371/journal.pone.0178203.

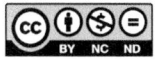

Index

© E. Fuller Torrey 2022
E. F. Torrey, *Parasites, Pussycats and Psychosis*,
https://doi.org/10.1007/978-3-030-86811-6